When Parkinson's Strikes Early

Advance Praise for *When Parkinson's Strikes Early*

"When Parkinson's Strikes Early *is a timely addition to guide books for people with Parkinson's disease, their spouses, care-givers, and families. It addresses the particular issues and concerns of young people with PD. Traditionally, PD has been been viewed as a disease of old people since the mean age of onset is 60 years. Recently, however, everyone has been struck by the 'epidemic' of young people that has been highlighted by the appearance of PD in Michael J. Fox. Young people with PD have special concerns: having children, raising a family, planning for the future. These concerns are addressed in this book. The book, however, is of interest to all people with PD and is recommended for anyone with PD, their spouses, care-givers, family, and friends.*"

—Abe Lieberman, M.D.
Medical Director of the National Parkinson Foundation

"...*your book truly put a face on this disorder and I thank you.*"

—Judith Horowitz, Ph.D.
Assistant Professor of Psychology and Parkinson's researcher, Medaille College

"*This work clearly demonstrates the tremendous impact of Parkinson's disease throughout the world and the urgent need for increased education for patients, caregivers and health care professionals. The book is unique in that it provides a patient perspective on living with Parkinson's disease. From the time of diagnosis throughout the course of the disease, it conveys the many emotional and physical changes that a person with Parkinson's disease experiences. It provides not only educational information, but more importantly validates the many emotions that persons with Parkinson's disease will encounter throughout their lives. This book would benefit any parkinsonian patient by providing access to a unique support system in which they can express their feelings, gain information and most importantly, be reassured that they are not alone.*"

—William C. Koller, M.D., Ph.D.
Director of Movement Disorders,
University of Miami Medical Center
National Research Director, National Parkinson Foundation

"*The material gathered by the authors makes an excellent book and one that I hope will be read by members of the multi-disciplinary teams involved with the treatment of people with Parkinson's. There is a wealth of experience and depth of understanding about living with the condition to be learned from this clearly laid out book.*"

—Emma Bennion
Chairman of YAPP&Rs, 1997–2000

"*Sourced from an impressive list of references, there are the 'classic' writings well known to those from PIEN as well as contributions from distinguished health professionals. The book weaves together accounts from over 70 young PIEN subscribers with timely medical facts and accurate analysis. Carefully selected, and never too long, the chapters flow seamlessly with the stories of those who have progressed down the Parkinson's pathway.*"

—Ms. Joy Graham, Western Australia

"*In 1990, when I was diagnosed with Parkinson's, there were practically no good books about the disease for the layman. That's no longer true, and* When Parkinson's Strikes Early *is one of the reasons. It is chockablock with not only information but also wisdom—the wisdom of experience. Its main characters, speaking to each other via the Internet, tell stories that are sometimes poignant, sometimes funny, often eloquent and—at their best—inspiring.*

—Joel Havemann
Reporter, L.A. Times

To the healers of the world.

Ordering

Trade bookstores in the U.S. and Canada please contact:
Publishers Group West
1700 Fourth Street, Berkeley CA 94710
Phone: (800) 788-3123   Fax: (510) 528-3444

Hunter House books are available at bulk discounts for textbook course adoptions; to qualifying community, health care, and government organizations; and for special promotions and fund-raising. For details please contact:

Special Sales Department
Hunter House Inc., PO Box 2914, Alameda CA 94501-0914
Phone: (510) 865-5282   Fax: (510) 865-4295
E-mail: ordering@hunterhouse.com

Individuals can order our books from most bookstores, from our website at
www.hunterhouse.com, or by calling toll-free:
(800) 266-5592

When Parkinson's Strikes Early

Voices, Choices, Resources, and Treatment

Barbara Blake-Krebs, M.A.

&

Linda Herman, M.L.S.

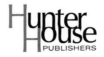

Hunter House
PUBLISHERS

Hunter House Inc., Publishers
PO Box 2914
Alameda CA 94501-0914

Library of Congress Cataloging-in-Publication Data
When parkinson's strikes early : voices, choices, resources, and treatment / by Barbara Blake-Krebs and Linda Herman.
p. cm.
Includes bibliographical references and index.
ISBN 0-89793-340-0 (pb)
1. Parkinson's disease—Popular works. I. Blake-Krebs, Barbara. II. Herman, Linda.
RC382 . W48 2001
616.8'33—dc21
2001016619

Project Credits
Cover Design: Peri Poloni, Knockout Design
Book Production: Michael Zipkin, Lucid Design
Developmental Editor: Rosana Francescato
Copy Editor: Kelley Blewster
Proofreader: John David Marion
Indexer: Kathy Talley-Jones
Acquisitions Editor: Jeanne Brondino
Associate Editor: Alexandra Mummery
Editorial and Production Assistant: Emily Tryer
Acquisitions and Publicity Assistant: Lori Covington
Sales and Marketing Assistant: Earlita K. Chenault
Publicity Manager: Sara Long
Customer Service Manager: Christina Sverdrup
Order Fulfillment: Joel Irons
Administrator: Theresa Nelson
Computer Support: Peter Eichelberger
Publisher: Kiran S. Rana

Printed and Bound by Bang Printing, Brainerd, Minnesota

Manufactured in the United States of America

9 8 7 6 5 4 3 2 1   First Edition   01 02 03 04 05

Table of Contents

Important Note

The material in this book is intended to provide a review of information regarding young-onset Parkinson's disease. Every effort has been made to provide accurate and dependable information. The contents of this book have been compiled through professional research and in consultation with medical professionals. However, health-care professionals have differing opinions, and advances in medical and scientific research are made very quickly, so some of the information may become outdated.

Therefore, the publisher, authors, and editors, and the professionals quoted in the book cannot be held responsible for any error, omission, or dated material. The authors and publisher assume no responsibility for any outcome of applying the information in this book in a program of self-care or under the care of a licensed practitioner. If you have questions concerning your nutrition or diet, or about the application of the information described in this book, consult a qualified health-care professional.

Foreword

On behalf of the all those who face the daily challenges of Parkinson's disease and the health-care professionals who try to help ease the burden, I offer a heartfelt thank you to Barbara Blake-Krebs and Linda Herman for undertaking the enormous project of producing *When Parkinson's Strikes Early*. They have compiled a unique book from the e-mail questions and responses of young people who joined the Parkinson's Information Exchange Network (PIEN) in search of information and support from others who are trying to cope with this disease. Barbara and Linda's sensitive editing and narration provide accurate and essential education and encouragement to anyone affected by this devastating, progressive neurological disorder. As a result of Barbara and Linda's vision and determination, the Parkinson's community now has a guidebook to illuminate the journey down the winding road of this complicated disease. What better guide on any journey than fellow travelers who allow us to learn from their stories and experiences? *When Parkinson's Strikes Early* gives voice and visibility to the thousands of young people who are struggling in the prime years of their life to deal with this "old people's disease."

As all of us working in this field know, there is very little in the literature that focuses on the younger patient. Even with the media coverage surrounding Michael J. Fox, most of the public still thinks of Parkinson's as an old person's disease and has very little knowledge about the disease in either the young or the old.

In my position as Coordinator of the American Parkinson Disease Association's National Young-Onset Information and

Referral Center, it is not uncommon to hear stories from young people, much like those presented here, describing puzzling early signs, worsening symptoms, and lengthy, circuitous routes to a correct diagnosis. It has been my experience that some physicians are still reluctant to make a diagnosis of Parkinson's disease in a young person, often stating to the patient, "Looks like Parkinson's, but you are too young to have it." For some young people, the diagnosis of Parkinson's disease comes as a relief. They finally have a name for the array of symptoms they are experiencing and confirmation that they are not crazy.

It is difficult for a person at any age to receive the diagnosis of this chronic progressive disorder, but to grapple with its impact at a young age is hardly imaginable. The future may seem jeopardized by uncertainties: "What can I expect? Will I be able to continue working? What kind of medical bills can I expect? Will I still be able to function as a nurturing parent and spouse?" The storytellers in this book address those challenging issues with practical information and support, not only about physical problems, but also about the unique social, family, and financial concerns that young people with PD must also face. From their multiple perspectives and experiences, they reach out to each other, offering answers, sharing resources, and providing encouragement. Many refer to the members of the PIEN as their "cyberspace family."

In our Center, over the years we have witnessed the positive value of direct person-to-person contact in supporting patients and their families. We have facilitated the development of Parkinson's support groups around the United States and we developed a Person-to-Person Network for those who prefer one-to-one contact rather than or in addition to a group. In addition, we created PDKIDS, an Internet forum for children to "talk" and to share questions and concerns when someone they love has Parkinson's. The storytellers in this book offer that same sense of intimate connectedness to someone who understands. The personal and often poignant voices of the storytellers in this book are representative of the voices of the over

2,000 people from more than 36 countries in this cyberspace support group—perhaps the largest Parkinson's support group in the world!

Bravo to Barbara and Linda who, despite their own struggles with this disease, have persevered to give us an "up-close and personal" understanding of Parkinson's disease, particularly in the younger person. It is a guidebook par excellence for anyone affected by Parkinson's disease. In addition to patients and their families, *When Parkinson's Strikes Early* will help educate both health professionals and the lay public about the disease and provide important lessons about facing life's challenges with courage, perseverance, and humor.

Susan Reese, MA, RN, LCSW
Coordinator, American Parkinson Disease Association
National Young-Onset Information and Referral Center

Acknowledgements

The power of community is one of the themes of *When Parkinson's Strikes Early*, and it is the force behind this book. During our 2½-year collaboration, we received assistance and encouragement from members of many communities—our families, friends, colleagues, publisher, Parkinson's organizations, and our local and cyber-support groups. We would like to thank them all and to especially acknowledge the following individuals who read parts of our manuscript at various stages of its development and shared with us their honest opinions, insights, and knowledge:

Ken Aidekman, Emma Bennion; "Betsy" Blake, Hilary Blue; Perry Cohen, Ph.D.; Charles D'Aniello; Rona D'Aniello; Jeanette Fuhr; Joy Graham; Ed Herman; Kathrynne Holden; Tomas Holmlund, M.D.; Judith Horowitz, Ph.D.; Celia Jones; Professor Frederick A. "Fred" Krebs; William F. Koller, M.D.; Abraham Lieberman, M.D.; Kelly Lyons, Ph.D.; Lupe McCann; Kathleen McWhorter, Ph.D.; Charlie Meyer, M.D.; Mary Rack; Susan Reese; Michael Rezak, M.D.; Alan Richards; Barbara Schirloff; Frada Steinhaus; Phil Tompkins; Margaret Tuchman; Evie Weinstein; Cheryl Werner; and Mary Yost.

We thank our publisher for recognizing the importance of our stories being told to a wide audience and for taking a chance on two first-time authors. Everyone at Hunter House has been enthusiastically supportive and patient, especially editors Jeanne Brondino and Alexandra Mummery. They probably learned more than they ever wanted to about PD—especially about its effects on meeting deadlines.

Most of the selections in this book originated on the Parkinson's Information Exchange Network discussion list (Parkinsn list). Our gratitude goes to its international team:

Barbara Patterson of Canada, the list's owner and moderator for creating this invaluable resource that has touched so many lives throughout the world;

Simon Coles of the United Kingdom, for volunteering his time and computer expertise for hosting and managing the Parkinsn list archives, as well as a number of other special interest and multilingual PD mailing lists and;

John Cottingham of the United States, for designing and administering the PIEN Online webpage, with its many "treasures" for those seeking information about the disease and easy access to the list's current messages.

Barbara Blake-Krebs would also like to individually thank these special people:

Professor A. J. "Jack" Langguth, author, for his immediate and steadfast support of this project, as well as for many hours years ago of letting me hone my verbal skills on his awesome closet of comic books.

My two "baby" brothers, Michael J. Blake, attorney, who encouraged me to the extent that he would personally print the book if necessary—it wasn't!—and Stephen R. Blake, wind energy expert, who is helping this coauthor have many additional personal resources towards recovery following additional health problems in March 2000.

My Dad and Mom (1918–2000), for their unfailing support through the years.

My husband, Frederick A. Krebs, a community scholar extraordinaire, who believes unwaveringly in me, challenges me, cares for me, and provides opportunities, tools, and most of all, love.

My coauthor, Linda Herman, and our mutual friend, Jeanette Fuhr, for choosing to include me in the initial brainstorming session on how we could raise public awareness and to trust me enough to collaborate. The initial 11 months it took

Linda and I to plan and produce the main draft (plus ensuing revisions) are among the most interesting and stimulating periods of my life. Their friendship and constant faith in the book have been great gifts, and I am so grateful for them.

Linda Herman adds special thanks to:

My family for their unfailing support and love and for understanding why I needed to devote so much of my time and attention to this project;

My children Michelle and Andy, who have grown into wonderful, caring, and intelligent adults and are the pride of my life;

My husband, Ed, who has always been there for me, and I know always will. I am truly blessed to have him as my partner in life;

My friends Barbara Blake-Krebs and Jeanette Fuhr for sharing this amazing experience with me, listening to my "Twilight Zone" stories, and believing in this project and in each other. And to Barb for her inspiring courage and determination in fighting her personal battle against Parkinson's disease.

Barbara Blake-Krebs, Merriam, Kansas
Linda Herman, Amherst, New York

Introduction

If nothing is real to medical researchers except as it
happens to a significant number of people, nothing is
real to a writer save as it happens to a single person.
NORMAN COUSINS[1]

IN DECEMBER 1998, popular actor Michael J. Fox stunned
the world by disclosing that he had been stricken with
Parkinson's disease (PD) at the young age of 30 and had
managed to hide his symptoms from the public for seven years.
When Representative Morris K. Udall, longtime United States
congressman from Arizona, passed away just a few days later,
the public was largely unaware that he had battled the same
disease for more than 20 years.

About Parkinson's Disease

Parkinson's is a degenerative, neurological disease of usually
undetermined origins, with no definitive diagnostic test (other
than autopsy) and no known cure. Its most common physical
symptoms include tremor (or shaking), stiffness, slowness of
movement, freezing (the inability to move), and poor balance.
Currently available medications often cause side effects within
5 to 10 years that can be worse than the disease symptoms
themselves, such as dyskinesia (uncontrollable movements).

Contrary to the common image of Parkinson's as a disease
of old age, PD can strike at any age, even during the teen years.
An estimated 15 percent of patients are diagnosed under the age
of 50, and the numbers are growing. The National Institute of

Neurological Diseases and Stroke predicts that until a cure is found, virtually everyone "will be touched by Parkinson's disease in some way, whether they develop the disease themselves or know someone else who is afflicted."[2]

Yet there is a scarcity of public knowledge and understanding about the disease and the people living with it. Their progressing immobility, ravaged voices, and frozen, expressionless faces (called Parkinson's masks) often keep them hidden—physically, emotionally, and intellectually—from the rest of society, and from one another. For many years, people with Parkinson's (PWPs) were also "invisible" to government officials who allocate funding for medical research, thus slowing the progress of Parkinson's research. It took a young lawyer with PD named Joan Samuelson, the discovery of the Internet as a tool for political activism, and a growing number of PWPs who vowed to be "Invisible No More" to transform isolated individuals into a strong, effective community of advocates.

About Our Storytellers

In this book, you will meet over 70 members of the Parkinson Information Exchange Network (PIEN), an international Internet discussion group. Our contributors come from many different countries, walks of life, and backgrounds, but they or their loved ones have all been diagnosed with Parkinson's "too early" in life. By sharing their stories, they hope to ease the journeys of those who follow and to raise public awareness about Parkinson's disease. Their selected e-mail messages to the PIEN, as well as other writings, have been woven together with accounts about Congressman Udall, Joan Samuelson, Michael J. Fox, and boxing legend Muhammad Ali into a unique global conversation about living with young-onset Parkinson's disease.

About the Authors

Barbara Blake-Krebs was a founder, administrator, and producer at community radio station KKFI-FM when she was diagnosed with PD in 1984, at age 44. She found a paucity of patient-oriented literature, but she was fortunate to locate a nearby Greater Kansas City–area support group that provided interaction with other PWPs and information about the elusive disease. However, during the early 1990s, progressing symptoms and weariness caused her to drastically reduce her involvement with the radio station and her other associations. She grappled with a growing state of dependency and isolation.

Ten years later, halfway across the country in Buffalo, New York, 45-year-old Linda Herman, a college librarian, was experiencing unusual but seemingly benign physical changes—her left foot dragged, her arm didn't swing naturally, her handwriting became small and cramped. Finally, when her left hand began to shake, she consulted her family doctor, who remarked, "You have all the symptoms of Parkinson's disease, but I've never seen it in somebody so young!" A neurologist later confirmed the uncertain diagnosis.

Linda was hungry for information about the disease, but also found very little comprehensive, nontechnical information from the patient's point of view, and even less from the unique perspective of the young-onset patient. She tried attending local Parkinson's support-group meetings and looked for others close in age, but found few peers. Like Barbara, she felt very alone with her new life's "companion." Finally, surfing on the Internet late one night, she accidentally discovered the Parkinson's Information Exchange Network, where she found the support and knowledge she had been seeking since her diagnosis.

Meanwhile, during her ensuing 10 years with PD, Barbara had become increasingly housebound. Her husband, Fred, encouraged her to learn some basic Internet functions, and she was soon happily able to expand her horizons online. The day in April (Parkinson's Awareness Month) 1996 when she joined PIEN was one of pure joy. Among the nearly 1,500 members from 36 countries, she found a highly nurturing community.

Since its founding in 1993 by Barbara Patterson of Ontario, Canada, PIEN has been crucial in breaking through the isolation and invisibility experienced by many people with Parkinson's.

In this virtual village, we (Barb and Linda) found acceptance, up-to-the-minute information, support, laughter, and sometimes tears. We became acquainted with PWPs from all over the world, including each other and Jeanette Fuhr of Missouri, the godmother of this book.

Why We Wrote This Book

Michael J. Fox's announcement served as a catalyst for our writing *When Parkinson's Strikes Early*, which was originally conceived as a letter to the editor to raise public awareness about young-onset PD. As we added the voices of other PIEN members to ours, the letter grew into an article, and finally we concluded, "Why not a book?" Jeanette encouraged our collaboration from the start, contributed her words, wisdom, and spirit, and cheered us on whenever we became discouraged.

Two years and hundreds of e-mail exchanges later, we believe our collaboration will fill a void in the literature about Parkinson's disease and promote understanding about coping with chronic illness of any kind. *When Parkinson's Strikes Early* offers patient-oriented information about physical symptoms at different stages of the disease and practical suggestions about coping with the changes and challenges PD brings into our lives. Additionally, the book examines the social and economic impact of young-onset PD on individuals, families, and society. PWPs, especially the newly diagnosed, will find much-needed understanding and information in these pages. Medical personnel and other professionals who work with Parkinson's patients will gain new insights into the realities of living with PD. The lessons learned by those in the Parkinson's community about cooperation and political activism may be inspirational and instructional to members of other advocacy groups.

Above all, we hope our readers will come away with the understanding that there is life after Parkinson's. It can be a devastating disease, indeed; however, by educating ourselves, taking an active role in treatment, seeking the support of others, and mostly by facing life with hope, we can meet the challenges. By working together as a community, we will beat this disease.

The authors, in hopes of bringing the end of Parkinson's disease a little closer, will donate all royalties from the sales of *When Parkinson's Strikes Early* to PD research and programs that improve the lives of PWPs. As we enter the twenty-first century, new treatment options are becoming available, and researchers now predict that a breakthrough is likely in 5 to 10 years. We are hopeful, yet still uncertain, about how our journeys will proceed and how they will end. In the words of Dennis Greene, one of our storytellers from Australia:

I didn't come here for this,
this endless journey on broken roads.
My route was planned over perfect highways
with scenic stopovers.
I knew where I was going.
No I didn't come here for this.[3]

Our journeys begin....

chapter 1

Welcome to the Journey

THE HONORABLE MORRIS "MO" K. UDALL served in the House of Representatives for 30 years, from 1961 to 1991, as a congressman from Arizona. He was known nationally as a dedicated advocate for environmental protection, a champion of social reform, and "the funniest man in U.S. politics." Mo's integrity and humanity earned him the respect of his colleagues from all shades of the political spectrum. He aspired to one day being elected to the White House.

The bicentennial year of 1976 marked Udall's entry into the Democratic primaries for president. It also was the year that his Parkinson's disease symptoms first appeared, at the age of 54. Mo appeared symptom-free in public until the early 1980s, when his stooping posture, tremor, speech problems, and "Parkinson's mask" became noticeable.

As the disease progressed and his symptoms worsened, Mo fell under increasing pressure to retire from the House of Representatives, but he chose to resist, preferring to remain working at a job he loved. When the *Arizona Republic* urged him to retire in 1989, Udall defended his decision to remain in Congress, writing about Parkinson's, "It is not a fun illness.... It makes me stiff and causes me to lose facial expression. I sometimes think it is a more painful disease for others to witness than it is for me to bear. It is a disease I will not die from, but will die with."[1] It was only after injuries from a fall brought on incapacitating disability that he resigned from office in 1991. By 1993, when Canadian Barbara Patterson founded the Parkinson's Information Exchange Network (PIEN), an international e-mail discussion group, Mo was confined to a VA hospital bed, unable to walk or talk. Though he was never able to join the global conversation taking place in the Internet Parkinson's community, PIEN members felt his presence. His example of facing PD with courage and advocating for issues he believed in inspired many. "Do it for Mo!" became the rallying call of a growing grassroots campaign for equitable funding for PD research. Learning the art of advocacy and collaboration, PWPs worked together as a politically active community for the first time and found that even weakened voices could be heard on Mo's Capitol Hill.

Thus, it is fitting to include Representative Udall's experiences with Parkinson's disease alongside those of PIEN members from around the world who, like Mo, were also stricken with Parkinson's "too early" in their lives.

Parkinson's Disease: The Basics

NANCY MARTONE, TEXAS How many times have you seen someone and thought, "Gee, he/she must have Parkinson's disease"? My guess is not too many. However, you may have seen someone who has a noticeable tremor in one or both hands, or who seems to shiver on the hottest of days.

Perhaps you've noticed that a friend's posture has changed and he's walking more slowly and looks rather "stiff." Or how about that man in the theater, the one who didn't crack a smile the whole evening, and just sat there? Well, guess what! You may have been seeing people with Parkinson's![2]

What Is It?

Parkinson's disease (PD) is a progressive neurological disease affecting certain cells in the middle part of the brain known as the substantia nigra, a control center for movement. Dopamine produced by these cells is the neurochemical messenger essential for smooth and normal movements. These cells degenerate and die in PWPs at a more rapid rate than in the general population. Many researchers believe that an interaction between a genetic predisposition and environmental factors may trigger early brain-cell degeneration. When the loss of those cells lowers the supply of dopamine below necessary levels, a garbling of nerve messages between the brain and the muscles occurs—causing the movement problems of Parkinson's disease. (See Chapter 8 for more about possible causes of PD.)

Although there are some similarities between the neurodegenerative disorders of Parkinson's and Alzheimer's diseases, in terms of effects on their victims, they are opposites. While Alzheimer's destroys the mind, leaving the body functioning, Parkinson's destroys the body's ability to function, imprisoning the mind inside.

How Many People Have It?

Due to the scarcity of epidemiological studies on Parkinson's disease, conclusive statistics are unavailable. However, the following estimates are generally accepted:[3]

- ▶ At least four million people throughout the world suffer from the disease.
- ▶ There are over one million people in the United States and over 100,000 in Canada diagnosed with Parkinson's disease.
- ▶ Each year 60,000 new cases are diagnosed in the United States.
- ▶ The average age of onset is about 55. PD affects about 1 percent of the population over age 55.
- ▶ Fifteen percent of all Parkinson's patients are diagnosed under the age of 50; 10 percent are under 40.
- ▶ The numbers of younger people diagnosed with PD are growing.

Dr. Donald Calne, a Parkinson's expert, states, "Parkinson's has been called the silent epidemic.... And it's a growing one. I have tracked Parkinson's patients for more than three decades, and have already seen a fourfold increase in younger patients."[4]

What Is Young-Onset PD?

The answer to this question depends on whom you ask. Some sources define young-onset as symptoms first occurring between the ages of 21 and 40. Others designate 45, 50, or 55 years of age as the cutoff point. Some definitions use the term "diagnosis" rather than "onset of symptoms." This is a significant difference, since it is common for younger patients to experience symptoms for many years before being diagnosed, and it is often difficult to know exactly when the symptoms began. Yet another statistical definition utilizes age 55, the average age of onset, as the cutoff for young-onset Parkinson's disease (YOPD).

Another method of defining YOPD is to consider the patient's life situation, rather than chronological age. The British organization YAPP&Rs (Young Alert Parkinson's Partners & Relatives) describes itself as a "special interest self-help group for people with Parkinson's and their families who are of working age and below."[5] This outlook recognizes that PWPs of any age who are raising children and/or working outside the home have unique concerns, interests, and needs. Finally, according to PIEN list member Anne Rutherford, her support group in Newfoundland, Canada, "…lets you be a young Parkie if you say you are."

Since this book examines many aspects of life with Parkinson's, we believe that a holistic definition, which encompasses all of the above, is the most appropriate.

Early Missed Diagnosis: The Mask of Youth

Young-onset Parkinson's patients often share stories about the misdiagnosis of their early symptoms. Parkinson's can be a difficult disease to diagnose. Physicians who are not well trained in neurological disorders often do not consider PD as a possibility in younger men and women, even when faced with the typical symptoms. We advise anyone experiencing movement problems such as those discussed later in this chapter, under the subhead titled "The Early Symptoms of PD," to seek evaluation by a neurologist who specializes in Parkinson's disease or movement disorders. Many of the PD organizations listed in the resource guide (Appendix 2) offer assistance in locating these specialists.

JEANETTE FUHR, MISSOURI Welcome to the journey of living with Parkinson's disease. It's a twisting road of adventure, challenges, and milestones strewn with the objects we discard or lose along the way: broken dreams, grand plans, mislaid notions. Fortunately, many traveled the road before and are willing to share their exploits, triumphs, and defeats with those just beginning the trail.

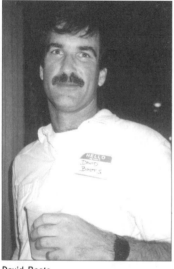

David Boots

DAVID BOOTS, CALIFORNIA I am David, 36 years old and diagnosed with PD for 4 years. Music is the brightest part of my life. I have been playing music since I was 13 years old, when I saw a kid about my age playing banjo on a local television show in Memphis. I've been hooked ever since.

I have won banjo and guitar contests, played in a variety of bands across the United States, and have taught (formally) at least 50 people how to play the guitar or banjo. Then came Parkinson's.

The symptoms of PD (first noticed in 1985) started to affect me significantly in 1988. At first, they were a nuisance, but I was still able to function well enough for the most part. I joined a bluegrass band and found that my late-night banjo playing had a new twist. As the evening wore on, my dexterity and speed were greatly reduced. My fellow band members were as confused as I was, since "David was playing fast just a while ago...what's up?" I also heard people remark, "You play the banjo really well, but you need to smile more." Not knowing then about the PD mask, I assured people that I was smiling inside (though it rarely made it to the outside of my face).

In 1988 I went to the hospital to ask about these peculiar physical traits. The doctor, who was not a neurologist, checked me out and informed me, "You're experiencing an isolated muscle tremor. They can come and go at any age. I wouldn't worry about it." That was a relief. An isolated muscle tremor I could handle![6]

RICHARD PIKUNIS, NEW JERSEY When I was 24 years old, my symptoms were apparent, but because of my age and general overall good health, I went undiagnosed.

I had the symptoms associated with a typical Parkinson's patient: slowness and loss of movement, postural instability resulting in frequent falls, a distorted gait and muscle rigidity. I remember not going on a family vacation because my body ached so badly and I was so stiff and rigid that walking consumed all my energy.

Because of a common misconception that Parkinson's disease is a geriatric disorder, the diagnosis wasn't as obvious as it should have been. Besides, I don't exhibit the most prominent, telltale symptom of Parkinson's—the tremor. In fact, according to the American Parkinson Disease Association (APDA), tremors only occur in about 70 percent of patients. It is usually the tremors that bring the patient to the doctor.[7]

LYNDA MCKENZIE, ONTARIO, CANADA I began to notice a slight trembling of my arm when it was at rest. Because my daughter is diabetic, I thought it could possibly be low blood sugar, so I started doing blood readings. They were, of course, normal. I looked up "tremor" in our home medical guide. The book said that at-rest tremor is a symptom of Parkinson's, but it also stressed that this only happens to people over 55. I happily shut the book on that option.

HILARY BLUE, SOUTH AFRICA/ISRAEL/VIRGINIA In 1976, I worked as a cataloguer/classifier in an Israeli medical school library. The head librarian loved my handwritten catalogue cards—because my writing was so tiny. But it was getting tinier and tinier, until he called me in one day to complain that it was so tiny as to be completely unreadable!

At the same time, my arm had this strange feeling of weakness, and I was beginning to drag my right leg. Field day for the medical school! Every doctor, every resident, and every intern had his own theory of what was wrong with me. I was diagnosed with mono, MS, polyarthritis, ankylosing spondylitis, pressure on a nerve in the neck. You name it, I had it, and had the treatment for it—none of which worked.

Meantime I also had a disastrous marriage, which shot through my life like a ball of exploding destruction. About my physical symptoms I was told, "It's the stress. When you calm down, it will go away."

JUDITH RICHARDS, ONTARIO, CANADA In the late 1980s, I noticed a weakness in my legs and a stiffness in my neck, but most of all, no matter how much sleep I got, a constant feeling of fatigue. I thought I had MS, but my family doctor told me I would have had symptoms at an earlier age. He ordered blood work, but nothing showed up, so I was left to carry on as though there were nothing wrong with me. Was it all in my head?

Over the next couple of years, I started experiencing severe migraine headaches, and any stressful situation sent me into fits of uncontrollable shaking. In 1991, my family doctor referred me to a neurologist. Diagnosis? Stress, and once again I was sent on my way.

JOHN QVIST, SWEDEN I have had very vague symptoms since I was 18 years old, but it was when I was 27 that the symptoms started to be troublesome. The stiffness in my left arm was joined by tremor. Since I work with computers, that was very annoying.

My first neuro told me (after a spinal tap and some blood work) that it was MS. My physiotherapist, though, said she could have sworn it was PD. When I told the neuro what my PT had said, the doc hesitated for a fraction of a second, then just shook her head.

JOHN BJORK, WEST VIRGINIA Before the PD was diagnosed, I suffered from unexplainable panic attacks stemming from worry about unresolved physical symptoms. I knew something was wrong, but the medical community marked it down as emotional. (My tombstone will read: "See, I told you I was ill.") I'm a 59-year-old male and was diagnosed with PD about 10 years ago. At first, when I heard that term, I thought it referred to someone from Parkinsaw (a fictional village).

JIM SLATTERY, AUSTRALIA The eventual diagnosis of my condition was complicated by the fact that I had had a bad motor accident shortly before I began noticing symptoms of PD. I was pursuing an insurance claim, which, before it was settled, resulted in my being referred by one side or the other in the claim to 27 different doctors, *none* of whom suspected or even hinted at PD. Most seemed to favor a psychological or psychiatric disorder.

I was 44 at the time, and I think that was a large part of the problem. Before about 1990, most health professionals were taught, in the wording of a popular medical text, that Parkinson's is "a disease of the sixth decade," in other words, of people 50 and over.

RICK BARRETT, CALIFORNIA I'm 34 years old. About 5 years ago I started getting some stiffness in my left hand, which made handwriting difficult. The docs at that time treated me for carpal tunnel syndrome. The thought was that I spent too much time on the computer—but I barely typed two pages a day. After 2 years of therapy and assorted meds, I was finally referred to a neurologist, who after a couple visits made the diagnosis—PD.

WILL JOHNSTON, MARYLAND The missed diagnosis of PD is horrendous. The internist I use said I might have PD, but he didn't think so. Two neurologists couldn't come up with PD. One seemed to think of nothing but the DTs (delirium tremens). The other just didn't know. I tried a chiropractor—the effect was an increase in the PD symptoms. I was scared he might have done something wrong and caused harm to me with his manipulations.

Why is the diagnosis of PD missed so often? One reason is the way medical schools teach. To teach the students about PD and how to recognize it, which PD patient does the professor show to his students? He picks the "best" one, the stage-four or -five case with all the symptoms, rather than the stage-one or -two patient who has years of problems ahead. Picking the worst

PD patient for the rounds is natural, but it is a disservice to the students and future patients.

JACQUELINE WINTERKORN, M.D., PH.D., CONNECTICUT/NEW YORK Why do I read exchanges among PD patients? Because as a physician I know that the only experts in a disease are the patients who have it.... Exchanges among PD patients and my own experiences have convinced me that there is a lot that is not taught and a lot that most physicians have not heard about this disease!

Unnecessary Surgeries and Treatments

One of the consequences of a missed diagnosis is that too commonly, young-onset PWPs are subjected to unnecessary and even potentially harmful therapies, medications, and surgery. Some are led to believe that the "problem is all in their heads" and are referred for psychological or psychiatric treatment. However, the "problems" facing these PWPs are the result of degeneration and death of their brain cells; they are not caused by emotional difficulties or an overactive imagination. By the time early symptoms of Parkinson's first become noticeable, it is estimated that 60 percent of nerve cells in the substantia nigra are already dead, and that 80 percent of their dopamine is lost.

SANDRA NORRIS, NORTH CAROLINA My first eight years of wrestling with PD were done in a psych's office, sometimes as inpatient, most of the time as outpatient. At the age of 20, my strange symptoms of left shoulder pain, tremor in left arm, unbalance, masked expression, panic attacks, body taking on 70-year-old shuffle step resulted in a diagnosis of "psychologically induced symptoms brought on to avoid facing life." At the age of 21, I endured the agony of three months in a psychiatric ward, where a neurologist who thought that being rude and blunt while examining me would "snap me out of behavior" allowed my tremor-ravaged body to slip onto the floor, saying "There is nothing wrong with you physically."

KEES PAAP, THE NETHERLANDS/TEXAS I was born on November 15 in Zandvoort, the Netherlands, during the best year after World War Two: 1949. I studied many evening hours, got married, became a daddy (daughter 18, son 15), and remained happy till March 1988. First I thought I had worked too hard and too much. My boss was very ill and I had to replace him, besides doing my own work. My GP [general practitioner] sent me to a neurologist who told me—after some tests—that I had carpal tunnel syndrome....

In November 1988, I returned to the neurologist because I could hardly use my hand. It gave me a lot of problems with writing and playing the trumpet. I had an unnecessary operation for carpal tunnel syndrome in December 1988 and was told it would be all better at the end of January. It became a little better.

BARBARA PATTERSON, ONTARIO, CANADA The first sign that anything was wrong with me was a sore shoulder. It continued for months, and nothing seemed to help it. X rays showed nothing wrong. Physiotherapy didn't help. Finally, I was referred to a rheumatologist, who gave me a cortisone shot in the shoulder (ouch!). The shoulder was better for a while.

The Early Symptoms of PD

Parkinson's is often called a "designer disease," because the symptoms vary so widely among individual patients. Some common early symptoms can include one or any combination of the following:

- ▶ tremor, usually with the limb at rest
- ▶ stiffness of arms, fingers, or legs
- ▶ dragging of leg(s) and unnatural swinging of arm(s) when walking
- ▶ low voice volume
- ▶ very small, cramped handwriting
- ▶ slow movement
- ▶ diminished sense of taste or smell
- ▶ difficulty swallowing

- ▶ internal tremor—inside the chest, abdomen, arms, or legs
- ▶ fatigue
- ▶ depression
- ▶ loss of facial expression—commonly called the Parkinson's mask

ANNE RUTHERFORD, NEWFOUNDLAND, CANADA It took a long time for the "whispers" of symptoms that I developed to be recognized as PD. I had no tremor at all. Doctors and others look for tremor, and if there isn't any, it isn't PD. The earliest symptom (10 years ago): left turns when skiing were not up to the same standard as right turns; putting in zippers became very difficult; it was hard to use power tools—my fingers and hands were clumsy and stiff.

I had a lot of shoulder pain; backing up the car was hard—I couldn't turn far enough as my neck was too stiff; immense fatigue; depression; I just sat; handwriting got smaller; lost my sense of smell. Ladies of 80 plus could walk faster than I could; my face became stare(y); when I swam lengths, I would fold up and sink without warning; I couldn't ride a bicycle any more because my balance was shot to hell.

These "symptoms" appeared very slowly—perhaps taking as long as seven years—and while I was upset that there was no apparent reason why I felt so dreadful most of the time, looking back, it was better not to know.

ALAN BONANDER, CALIFORNIA I am 53 [in 1994] and have been diagnosed with PD since 1984. My first symptoms started about 5 years earlier, when I was 38, with tremor in the left arm. Slowly I started to drag my left leg, and my left arm was not swinging when I walked.

JANE BONANDER (Alan's wife) His first symptoms went back as far as 1978 when he discovered a weakness in his left arm and leg, which he basically ignored.

BLAIR ASHWORTH, UNITED KINGDOM My symptoms first appeared about two years ago. Before then I had always suffered from stiff joints, and I was forever cracking my hands,...but I just thought they were symptoms of getting older. Then I noticed that my left arm was shaking, and my left leg started to drag as

I walked, but I ignored the signs.... To be frank, I was too frightened to admit that something might be wrong. I kept my feelings to myself for about a year, but during the spring of 1997 my arm wasn't doing what it should and I told my wife, Jill.[8]

JACQUELINE WINTERKORN I saved the consultation letter written 10 years ago by the first neurologist I contacted to confirm my self-diagnosed PD. Among my major complaints summarized in that letter was "a feeling of internal tremor." This bothered me especially in social situations, where I found it distracting. He concluded that I did not have PD—my diagnosis was not confirmed until a year (and two neurologists) later. Hearing about this symptom from so many others is heartening.

ANNE RUTHERFORD Re: masked face. I remember my mother used to have a blank look many years before her PD showed.
My kids say I did the same long before I was diagnosed.

TIM HODGENS, PSYCHOLOGIST, MASSACHUSETTS Clinically, the professional community deals with it by objectifying it and classifying it as "masked facies." Parkinson's disease is a disorder of both movement and expression. We are talking about having "lost" our face, or at least the use of it, which we had taken for granted. The face which we present to the world. The face which everyone notices.

JOAN SNYDER, ILLINOIS Unlike Zorro or poker players, we mere humans depend on our faces to convey our true feelings: to take the sting out of a reprimand, to show our concern and sympathy, to say, "I love you." This part of my disease is very hard for me to deal with. I used to be a bartender in my previous life (BPD—before Parkinson's disease), and I must admit that I could tell a joke or a story with the best of them. I had a strong, expressive voice and a kind of "Jim Carey" face to go along with it! My other vanity was my handwriting—everyone commented on what a lovely hand I had. I guess this must be God's way of teaching me humility—kind of like being a Cubs fan.

TIM HODGENS The "mask" is exactly that: a mask. It has little to do with the person inside. We must accept that radically. The person who does not runs the risk of becoming totally anonymous to the world. Do not let that happen.

LYNDA MCKENZIE The year was 1987. My children were 12 and 10, my crafts store was very busy, and I was dating a caring and exciting man. Not a bad year, except perhaps for a slight ache in my right leg when driving. Funny, things seemed to take longer to get done. Why was I getting so tired so quickly? My glue gun had become more difficult to use. What was happening?

My handwriting was hardly legible; checks were just as bad. I noticed that my right arm was slightly swollen and discolored.

On the phone and in my store, people often didn't hear what I said and would ask me to repeat myself. As far as I was concerned, they just weren't listening.

My aunt started working with me in the store as Christmas approached. I put everything down to stress, and the arm problem I assumed was carpal tunnel syndrome. I just didn't have the time for an operation and to sit around with my arm in a cast waiting for it to heal, so I didn't go to my doctor.

IVAN SUZMAN, MAINE By 1986, when my young-onset Parkinson's disease symptoms made their first appearance, I had 10 years of scholarly life behind me. I was publishing and at the beginning of a promising career as a research scientist, teacher, and a budding palaeoanthropologist. I was working closely with South African exiles in the United States and developed a unique collection of rare films, now housed at Bowdoin College, that document the secret popular resistance movement against South Africa's apartheid government from approximately 1956 through 1992. My life was the exciting world of fossil digs in Kenya, Ethiopia, and South Africa. Travel plans for Africa were continuously on the front burner.

One day, in September, 1986, I noticed that my right arm didn't swing while I was out in my neighborhood for my usual evening walk. My shoulder ached terribly, and my right arm just hung limply. I had to slap it with my left hand to move it.

The following May, I was swimming with some friends. On the way across the lake waters, while swimming a lazy, comfortable crawl stroke, my right arm simply stopped. I had a few panicky moments, my heart racing and pounding. I was afraid I might drown. I couldn't free my right arm from the pressure of the water. Had I not been very close to the shore, I could have been in trouble, because I also was suddenly cold and shivery.

Other early, unidentified symptoms were intractably stiff right back and shoulder blade muscles, foot cramps, toe curls in bed at night, stiffened wrist and hand joints, and sleep disturbances. These were all warning signs. Strangely, I had virtually no tremor.

HILARY BLUE It was in 1973 when I was 23 that I first noticed the tremor. I remember that quite clearly and can pinpoint it exactly, because in all other respects I was in tiptop condition. I had just been promoted to branch manager—the youngest in the Johannesburg (South Africa) Public Library. We used to all go out and eat lunch together. I would order a grilled cheese sandwich, because I could eat that with my hands and would not be embarrassed by the others seeing the food fall off my fork!

My piano playing was at its peak performance level. I had been the featured soloist in a recital, the only nonmusic graduate to be asked to perform. I had started taking singing lessons. Then I started having these "holes" in my voice. I'd be singing a song, or a scale, or an exercise, and suddenly my voice would vanish. Instant laryngitis, as it were. Nobody could explain it then, but now I suspect it had something to do with PD. It's as if my vocal chords would freeze for a couple of seconds.

Describe the Pain: Stanza One
RITA WEEKS

The wafting song of the lone flute,
The melody that once flowed when I touched the ivory keys,
the power of the crescendo,
all of these are silent now.
Today, a staccato high C announces each step
from the ankle junction of my brace.
Does it hurt? Describe the pain.
Would you ask again, if I did complain?

"But I'm Too Young": Getting the Diagnosis

The diagnosis of PD relies on clinical observations and medical tests such as MRI and blood tests are used to rule out other brain disorders. Doctors look for four cardinal signs:

- ▸ tremor or shaking in the limbs (usually when at rest)
- ▸ rigidity of the muscles
- ▸ bradykinesia (slowness of movement)
- ▸ postural instability (falling or imbalance when changing position)

However, these symptoms may also be indicative of a number of other disorders, and the reliability of diagnosis depends heavily on the training and clinical observation skills of the examining doctor. Some neurologists prescribe a trial with L-dopa (an artificial dopamine replacement) to see if symptoms improve. Currently, the only definitive method of confirming a diagnosis is by microscopically examining the brain at autopsy, revealing physical evidence of neuron loss and the telltale presence of Lewy bodies. These are abnormal protein collections that accumulate within the substantia nigra region of the brains of PWPs and are believed to be related to movement dysfunction.

Studies of autopsy results reveal that about 25 percent of PD diagnoses are incorrect.[9] It has also been estimated that for every diagnosed PWP, there is another one undiagnosed. Future advances in neuroimaging techniques should improve the accuracy of diagnosis and allow earlier detection.

BOB MARTONE, NANCY MARTONE'S HUSBAND, TEXAS The tremor is often described as "pill rolling." Imagine holding an aspirin between your thumb and index finger and trying to roll it back and forth between those fingers.

Rigidity might be described by imagining yourself in a full-body cast or by imaging your flexor muscles tightening so much that your spine begins to curve. The Latin words for these two phenomena are *paralysis agitans*—a paralysis of controlled body movement combined with an agitated uncontrolled movement of the limbs and head. (Kind of like a car stuck in neutral that has a misfiring spark plug.)

The slowness of movement is often accompanied by a masked facial expression and a softening of the voice. Until recently, these conditions—tremor, rigidity, and slowness of movement (and postural instability)—were about the only symptoms physicians could observe before making their diagnosis.

Another method doctors have relied on for confirming their diagnosis is observing how the patient responds to drugs used to treat Parkinson's symptoms—that is, do the drugs help?

Experiences of Diagnosis

The exact circumstances of receiving the news that one has an incurable degenerative disease is commonly remembered down to the littlest detail. Doctors can help their patients cope with the diagnosis by being truthful about the prognosis, encouraging patients to educate themselves, prescribing appropriate support services and therapies, and offering hope for the future.

EMMA BENNION, UNITED KINGDOM Receiving the diagnosis of Parkinson's disease is often a major challenge and trauma. How one is served the "life sentence" will form the way to how the patient with Parkinson's disease will respond in the future. I call it a "life sentence" because…until the cure is found, there will be limited parole. The moment of diagnosis is never forgotten and is often talked about…amongst PWPs. In my case, having been told there was nothing wrong with me and that it was my age, my hormones, etc., my diagnosis or "life sentence" became a personal battle!

Firstly, I had to prove there was something wrong with me and then show that I would not only survive, but that I could and would come out stronger. So the journey began, and…I set out on a road of discovery.[10]

DAVID BOOTS In 1990, I went back [to the hospital]. The doctor who saw me said, "I'm not a neurologist, but that looks like Parkinson's…but you're awfully young to have Parkinson's!" (This remark would be repeated many times from that point on.) After seeing one of their two neurologists and going through the exam, MRI, etc., my journey began.[11]

JEANETTE FUHR When my mobility was affected with a "frozen" shoulder that wouldn't even swing during my daily walks, I figured a quick trip to my M.D. and a shot of cortisone would fix me up pronto.

Two shots later and an MRI on my shoulder, elbow, and wrist that showed no reason for the pain/stiffness led to a referral to a neuro who said, "You might have Parkinson's, except at 47, you're too young."

But another MRI, this one on my head, showed no tumor, no stroke...and my identity as a PWP and a newbie (newly diagnosed PWP) began. I asked questions, I cried, I prayed, I asked my friends, church, and family to pray, I took drugs that my neuro prescribed, I asked for a second opinion from a movement-disorder specialist—and the diagnosis remained constant. I, however, have changed.

IVAN SUZMAN In 1989, I started losing control of pens and pencils. Handwriting started to be a problem. My arm muscles were not strong enough to push a ballpoint pen across a piece of paper. I had to quit my evening office job because of unbearable pain in my right arm. No one knew what was happening to me.

During the latter part of March 1989, when my left leg and foot seemed to be strangely weak and I kept stumbling and catching my left foot dragging, I decided to see a local neurologist. He diagnosed me with "Parkinson's Disease—30 years too soon."

He told me that I would do best to uproot myself and head for a warmer climate and that I must start medication immediately. I went into anger, frustration, and denial for 3 months.

BLAIR ASHWORTH My GP came to see me when he received test results eliminating other causes for my symptoms.... I remember sitting on the sofa in our front room, and my initial reaction was: "It can't be—I'm too young." I'd never heard of anyone under 60 having Parkinson's.[12]

BARBARA PATTERSON A year later I went back to the rheumatologist, this time with a sore shoulder and a sore knee, both on the left side. He decided it was time to get to the bottom of this and sent me to a neurologist who had her own series of tests for me. In September 1992, I was diagnosed with Parkinson's. Further tests eliminated other causes, so I was still diagnosed with Parkinson's.

ALAN BONANDER I eventually had five CAT scans, plus an MRI, evoke test, spinal tap, and cervical myelogram. When nothing showed, the neurologist said I had PD.

HILARY BLUE My new husband, Burt, put his foot down. "You can't go on living like this. You have to be there for the baby." Fighting words to an expectant mother. So off we went on a round of the doctors again, ending up at a neurologist, who stated categorically, "There is nothing wrong with you that a little rest and relaxation won't cure."

And then a few days later, I went along with Burt to meet his psychiatrist. The man had trained in England as a neurologist before specializing as a psychiatrist. He shook hands with me and said not "How do you do" but "Have you ever been tested for Parkinson's?" He had recognized the one symptom that nobody else had even looked for—the cogwheel effect in my wrist joints!

Now the doctors had a tentative diagnosis to confirm or deny. I did a whole battery of tests—including a spinal tap and CAT scan 18 months later—which showed absolutely nothing— of course. By now, when I was pregnant with my second child, the doctors had come to the reluctant conclusion that I had Parkinson's.

JACQUELINE WINTERKORN Today is my 50th birthday. I am a practicing M.D. and also have a Ph.D. in neurobiology and behavior. I have a busy practice, specializing in neuro-ophthalmology. I have had PD for a decade. I diagnosed myself, and the diagnosis was contradicted by the first two colleagues who examined me, but finally corroborated.

KEES PAAP At the end of April, I still had problems. So I went back to my neurologist. He was on vacation. His colleague told me—5 minutes after I entered his room—that he thought of Parkinson's. He did some simple tests, and five minutes later he told me that he was convinced I had Parkinson's disease. It was confirmed by a professor, and then I was certain.

I started to read about it. Pictures of elderly people, stories about elderly people. I became a member of the Dutch PD society and saw elderly people everywhere. In April 1992, I visited a meeting where I met some young people. I found out that I was not unique! I was very glad to find other young-onset PWPs.

JUDITH RICHARDS In February of 1993, after the death of my sister with whom I was very close, all the symptoms became worse. I was experiencing stiffness in other areas of my body, dragging my right foot, and the least little thing brought forth a flood of tears. Once again, I was referred to a neurologist, but because specialists are busy, it would be 6 months before I could see him.

So I started reading anything and everything I could get my hands on relating to the symptoms I was experiencing. By the time I saw the neurologist in August, I knew I had Parkinson's.

RICHARD PIKUNIS After years of knowing something was wrong but not quite able to put my finger on it, my mind was finally put at ease when the doctor told me I had Parkinson's. Yes, at the ripe old age of 27 years, and after three medical opinions, it was conclusive—I did have Parkinson's disease.

I was just starting out in life. The same age as my friends who were getting married and buying houses. They were enjoying life as I felt life was slowly being drained from my body.

Not knowing what Parkinson's was is probably why I wasn't as upset as my parents upon hearing the diagnosis. I remember my mother abruptly leaving the doctor's office, only to find her moments later in the car sobbing.[13]

LYNDA MCKENZIE A coworker, after seeing the state of my handwriting, told me that if I didn't go to my doctor right away, she would drag me to hers. When the doctor saw me, he made an appointment with a local neurologist. I asked my aunt to go with me. I had at last confided in her that I was sure I had carpal tunnel syndrome. I felt that if she came with me, she could listen to the doctor tell me that I needed an operation, and perhaps catch any details I might miss.

I remember the day well. May, the Friday before the long weekend, very hot, sunny, a beautiful day as we drove to Burlington, chatting about how we would manage with my arm in a cast. I wore my favorite pink pantsuit, because we planned to go shopping and have lunch after the appointment. When the doctor took me into the examining room, I honestly had no idea that within the next 45 minutes my future as I imagined it would be permanently altered.

BLAIR ASHWORTH I just assumed that I'd be given drugs and it would get better. That relief was short-lived. I didn't know much about Parkinson's at the time but the gradual realization that it was incurable and that treatments only controlled the symptoms—they didn't cure it—was devastating.

That's when panic set in.... I thought:

This can't be happening to me—not now, when I've got a young family to support. Why can't it go away and come back when I'm 55?[14]

Starting Down a New Path: Reactions and Changes

Receiving the news that one has a chronic, progressive neurological disease is a life-altering event at any age. Learning to accept the diagnosis and to face life with this unwelcome, ever-present companion often brings about deep reexamination of one's life vision, priorities, and relationships.

IVAN SUZMAN My diagnosis was confirmed in June 1989, by a neurologist in Boston. He told me that the best I could hope for was to attempt to mask the disease. There was no cure. For the 3 months that had passed after initial diagnosis, I had held off taking levodopa, the prescribed medication. After Boston, I knew I was an unusually early victim of a terrible and ugly disease. Only then did I try the medication the doctor had recommended—I had to accept the news.

JUDITH RICHARDS I started taking levodopa, the gold-standard drug for Parkinson's. I took a couple of months off work to get the diagnosis under my belt, and I joined the young-onset support group in London. After a couple of very tearful meetings, I settled into a life with my uninvited guest.

MARY YOST, CALIFORNIA The jolt of the diagnosis required me to put other aspects of my life in perspective and to "shape up or ship out." This is really no different than what my brothers both went through when they learned about their heart diseases, also when they were in their forties. They had to switch gears quickly, making some drastic lifestyle changes. When I compliment them on it, they say they really had no choice. Always unspoken is the "S" word. It's not an alternative, especially while we have kids who seem to still need us and while we have "miles to go before" we "sleep."

EMMA BENNION We need to hold onto as normal a life as possible. We need a positive attitude to PD and to take control of it as much as we can. I was to discover that being positive about PD helped open doors to people with further knowledge of the disease, which in turn helped me to "direct" my illness and to realize that life could go on.[15]

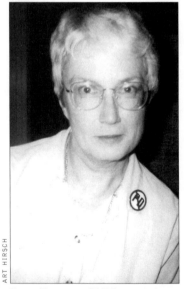

ART HIRSCH

Nancy Martone at PAN Forum

NANCY MARTONE PD is a challenging illness that affects both you and your family, but with faith in God, love and understanding of family and friends, and with hope for better treatments, or even a cure in the near future, we go on doing our best to smile and talk and lead as normal a life as possible.[16]

DENNIS GREENE, AUSTRALIA As for many others, that moment of diagnosis was for me one of those when the world shifts on its axis, and nothing will ever again be quite what it was or where it was before.

The problems that had taken me to the doctor in the first place were, it seemed, so minor—a cramped hand and a stiff arm—that my wife, Jo, had not accompanied me to the appointment. It was to be a few hours yet before she got to hear that "care-er" had been added to her job description and that her world too was moving in strange new ways.

For what it's worth, we spent the first couple of years after diagnosis swinging between denial and sheer terror. That stage does pass and will pass. I must admit, however, that I can still turn a corner in my mind and be ambushed by terror. Fortunately, these tend to be hit-and-run raids which don't last long.

How Barbara Patterson Came to Be a "List Mom"

When she was diagnosed, Barbara Patterson knew nothing about Parkinson's, nor anyone who had it, and little about computers. She had no inkling in November 1993 about the impact of her decision to start a Parkinson's support group on the Internet.

BARBARA The neurologist prescribed a medication twice a day and said to come back in a year. I read every book about Parkinson's that I could find. (A faculty member where I work suggested that I only read books published within the last few years.) I didn't know anyone with Parkinson's.

I went to one support-group meeting locally and decided it was not relevant to me. (It scared the daylights out of me!) I had joined a discussion list on the Internet called NURSENET, owned and operated by Judy Norris.

A friend of Judy's, Rina, was walking her dog in a park in Toronto and met a woman named Margret, who was also walking her dog. Margret has Parkinson's and during their conversation asked Rina if there was a discussion list on the Internet about Parkinson's. Rina asked Judy. Judy couldn't find one and posted a message to NURSENET asking about one.

I replied that I would join if she found one. Judy suggested (pushed, prodded, and urged) that I start one with her help. So we put together a proposal for the University of Toronto. They approved the proposal, and on 8 November 1993, away we went! Judy posted the new-list announcement in several places on the Internet, and we started to grow.

My purpose in starting the Parkinson List was the exchange of information about Parkinson's. The list rapidly changed into the largest support group I know. Besides its original purpose, the list has become a means of feeling connected to other members…a way of feeling we're not alone…of making life with PD easier to bear.

For more about PIEN, see Chapter 6.

Advice to the Newly Diagnosed

PHIL TOMPKINS, NEW JERSEY/MASSACHUSETTS   You learned that you have Parkinson's disease. You may have had any of a number of reactions—anxiety, disbelief, depression, fear, relief, a sense of loss, a sense of injustice, or something else. You may have wanted to cry on someone's shoulder or you may have wanted to be left alone.

You must have questions about what happens next and what you can do. That's a good sign. Your life is not going to proceed as you may have hoped, but your situation is far from hopeless. You will eventually face some limitations, but, because Parkinson's disease (PD) progresses slowly, you will have time to prepare for coping with further developments. And every few years there will likely be some new and more effective medicine.

It is possible to maintain a positive attitude. Since the time when I was diagnosed, I have had to stop working before I wanted to, and I can no longer play the piano—something I had planned to enjoy when I retired. My medicines don't work as well as they did at the beginning, and side effects can be as bad as the disease. But a number of good things have happened which would not have occurred otherwise, and for that I am grateful. Foremost among them is that I have met some truly wonderful people. My life is different, but it is no less rich.[17]

From Uninvited Guest to Master of the House: Symptoms and Side Effects as Parkinson's Disease Progresses

Never a Thought
MARVIN GILES

I never gave it a thought.
Getting up in the morning.
Going to bed at night.
Such simple things,
until you have to think about them.
Each act a battle of forced action.
Each detail a test of will.
Each motion an uncertainty.
Will I try today, or will I not?
I did try, and though the tears
fell like rain, I was successful
one more time.

The Process of Loss Begins

As the following discussions illustrate, the course of the disease's progression, the occurrence and severity of symptoms, and the response to medication can be quite different for each individual. Generally, in young-onset patients, the disease's progression tends to be more gradual than in those stricken later in life. Eventually, though, we become increasingly aware of PD's toll on our bodies and the limitations it imposes on everyday activities, even though our symptoms may remain unnoticeable by others.

NANCY MARTONE, TEXAS With PD, you are on a roller-coaster ride—one that never stops but just keeps encountering steeper climbs and deeper plunges. And as with a roller-coaster ride, it takes a long time to get to the top, you're only there for a second, and back down you go hitting that low spot faster and harder than before.

How do PWPs deal with the constant changes going on in their bodies? Well, there's always denial. That's a good way to start.

But all too soon, you can't ignore the tremor, or the rigidity, or the masklike expression you catch on your face when you glance in a mirror. You can't fool yourself that people aren't staring at your trembling hands as you look through your wallet or try to put together a bunch of papers.

So what do you do? Well, if you're lucky, you will be put on levodopa—that can be a real blessing, almost completely eliminating all symptoms…for a while.[1]

ANNE UDALL, DAUGHTER OF MORRIS K. UDALL The diagnosis of Parkinson's disease marked a major time in Dad's life and in the lives of those of us closest to him. I believed him to be invincible, unmarked by scandal as much as by time. I watched, at first with shock and dismay, as the daily routines of life became more difficult for him. And I wondered if he would give up. He didn't.[2]

JEANA BARTLETT, GEORGIA Your progression might be very slow. For me it was 8 years after diagnosis before the symptoms were so visible that everyone knew I had *something*! When I told them I'd had it for 8 years, they were shocked. I never doubted I had it...it just wasn't clamoring for my attention as it does now. It was like a "visitor" that came in and out of my life. Now it is the "master of the house"! It demands my attention.

Everyone is different. We hear that all the time, but no two persons follow the same pattern...at least I have seen this. It may be several years more before you experience worsening symptoms, and then again you may never.

LINDA HERMAN, NEW YORK I was diagnosed 5 years ago, and I continue to work full-time. I started a new job last year, and I did not reveal my condition until a year later, when I felt more confident that the truth would not jeopardize my position. My coworkers were surprised by my announcement. No one had noticed any of my symptoms—even though I thought they were becoming apparent. My friends tell me I look the same. I appreciate every day I can continue to lead my "normal" life. You learn what is really important.

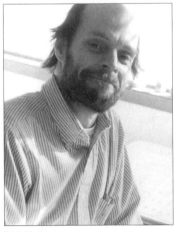

Rick Hermann

RICK HERMANN, WASHINGTON I was thinking about terminology yesterday and came up with the idea of being "less-abled" rather than "disabled," since I'm not the latter. I still go to work, ride a bike, and do lots of things. But I do less, and I do them less well. PD has caused in me a diminishing of capabilities, but not, so far, their disappearance. So I guess I have a lessability.

BLAIR ASHWORTH, UNITED KINGDOM I have to accept that my condition will get progressively worse and that my wife ...will be my main support. I just hope that medical advances will be such that there will be a cure for Parkinson's in my lifetime.... But that's all in the future. I'm managing for now and that's what's important.[3]

As the Disease Progresses...

Parkinson's is constantly on the offensive, destroying more and more dopamine-producing brain cells, as it marches on. Until a cure is found, PWPs are faced with a life of ever-evolving physical changes, choices, and challenges.

NANCY MARTONE As the disease progresses, you find yourself having to give up some things. Sometimes, it may be simply a matter of priorities. As you tend to have good times or "on" times as we call them, and bad times or "off" times, you have to decide what you have to do or want to do and let go of that which can wait or be ignored. Sometimes you are fortunate in that what you have to give up is something you didn't like doing anyway. One thing I found easy to give up was peeling potatoes. Giving up golf and tennis was a different story.[4]

JIM CORDY, PENNSYLVANIA I have witnessed this disease slowly but surely erode my physical abilities. I can no longer tie my tie, wash my hair or tuck my shirt in. I can't shuffle papers or drive my car. I have lost my facial expression, sense of smell, and I now have a monotone voice.[5]

STAN HOUSTON, TEXAS After a few years you realize your entire life has changed. Even the little things. Not long ago, my first priority before leaving the house was to make certain my wallet and keys were securely stuffed inside my jeans pocket. Who cares about credit cards and cash? Don't let me out the door without at least three emergency doses of pills.[6]

SANDRA NORRIS, NORTH CAROLINA Why does the PD affect each one of us differently? By "differently" I mean difference in severity, difference in symptoms, and finally difference in the speed of progression. I am going into my 19th year with this disease. I almost feel guilty for being as well as I am. Yes, without my medication I would be in critical-care nursing, but with my medicines I manage fairly well.

NANCY MARTONE If nothing else PWPs have a lot of symptoms that are combined in a variety of ways and change during the progression of the disease. I call it the "Jekyll and Hyde Syndrome."

A PWP can be two entirely different people, sometimes in a matter of minutes. I can go from being completely self-sufficient and busy to completely immobile, incapable of getting up out of a chair or walking across a room. This is hard not only on me but also the family. Who am I going to be? Dr. Jekyll or Mrs. Hyde? Even I don't know.7

Describe the Pain: Stanza Two
RITA WEEKS

Stitches march in even rows across the threads of time.
Painted petals, twisted tendrils, shadow and sunlight
delicate shading from paynes grey to titanium white
as they brush kissed the surface
and skipped on to the next flower
But today, twist ties and cellophane present a challenge
Does it hurt? Describe the pain.
Would you ask again if I did complain?

Drugs in the Battle with PD: A Double-Edged Sword

There is currently no cure for Parkinson's disease. Medications are prescribed to help relieve the symptoms and attempt to slow the progression of the disease.

The most widely used PD medication is levodopa (L-dopa), known by a variety of brand names in different countries. Nearly everyone diagnosed with PD will eventually use a form of levodopa, which stimulates the remaining brain cells to produce more dopamine, and for most people works very well for the first few years. However, over time, levodopa can lose its effectiveness, requiring increasingly larger doses, and often causes side effects such as "on-off" fluctuations and dyskinesia (described later in this section), which can be as disabling as the PD symptoms themselves.

Neurologists agree that drug therapy should be started when symptoms begin to interfere with daily activities, although there is some disagreement about which medication to start at that time. Many recommend delaying levodopa in younger patients, instead turning to dopamine agonists (such as ropinerole, pramipexole, and pergolide). Levodopa may be added later. Another class of drugs, called COMT inhibitors (entocapone and tolcapone), which help levodopa work more efficiently, may also be added to the mix.

It is not in the scope of this book to provide in-depth descriptions of the many medications currently used by Parkinson's patients. Appendix 2 contains some excellent resources for such information. There are, however, three basic facts of life with PD:

1. Drugs become a central (and sometimes the central) concern in our lives.

2. Medications and dosage schedules must be carefully adhered to and may need to be adjusted fairly often. Determining optimal dosages tends to be based on trial and error and is different for each PWP. It is important for patients and doctors to work together to determine the most effective drug therapy.

3. Currently available medications do not cure PD, and at some point in the disease's progression, they will fail and other options will need to be considered.

RITA WEEKS, NEBRASKA The impact of chronic degenerative disease on a family is much greater than we imagined. We are aware of not only my gradual loss of movement, but more important, the loss of our freedom to plan. Plans for today and tomorrow include the three of us: Don, Rita, and Drugs…and the drugs have the deciding vote always.

HILARY BLUE, SOUTH AFRICA/ISRAEL/VIRGINIA My very first contact with the support-group network led to my seeing a movement-disorders specialist. This was a very fortunate meeting. She was immersed in PD research and quite appalled at the treatment I had allowed myself to be getting—not knowing any better. That I was overmedicated, that it was impossible to know which of the medications was causing which reaction—I was bloated and my legs were swollen, I had severe migraines several times a week, my legs were mottled and I had either tingling or no feeling at all over most of my limbs. She took me off everything except one drug, and most of those terrible side effects disappeared.

RICHARD PIKUNIS, NEW JERSEY I wake up every morning barely able to move until my medication kicks in. I am currently taking L-dopa to replace the dopamine that my body can no longer produce, but it is becoming less effective at the current dosage. I know L-dopa will not be able to adequately treat my symptoms forever.

It really scares me when I think about how my life will be in a few years if we don't find a better treatment or cure for Parkinson's. I wonder if I will be able to teach my children how to ride a bike or dance at their weddings. I am scared about forced retirement before I am financially stable. I just graduated from law school; believe me, I can't afford not to work. But I know the choice may not be mine to make, because with an increase in L-dopa comes debilitating side effects, such as involuntary body movements and motor fluctuations. Sometimes the side effects are just as bad as the disease.[8]

Parkiespeak—On/Off

It confounds the onlooker every time—one minute the other person speaks and acts naturally—the next minute his voice may dim, his body may grow stiff, tremor, or gyrate, and his face take on a blank expression. This sudden transition, called on/off in Parkiespeak, may for many become noticeable 5 to 10 years after being diagnosed.

DENNIS GREENE, AUSTRALIA "On" and "Off" in Parkiespeak refer to whether or not your body is responding to your PD medications (especially the levodopa meds). Not everybody experiences the on/off syndrome; some PWPs seem to level out and maintain a plateau. Others experience the on/off syndrome from the first, and a great many develop it as the disease progresses.

In short:

Off

1. The medications are not being effective.

2. PD symptoms predominate.

3. The PWP is slow, freezes, is prone to fall, has tremor, experiences rigidity, etc.

4. The severity of the PD symptoms varies from mild to extreme depending on the stage to which the disease has progressed.

On

1. The medications are being effective.

2. The PWP moves more freely (hence the association of "on" with movement); tremor and rigidity are significantly reduced.

3. As the disease progresses, the "on" periods tend to shorten and can involve medication-related side effects.

DAVID BOOTS, CALIFORNIA You know you're really off when:

▶ The mention of childproof caps brings a disconcerting feeling.

▶ You realize that you are a much better listener than you'd ever imagined.

▶ You struggle for many minutes trying to get your hand in your pocket to grab your house keys, only to discover that your hand has grown to immense proportions and seems to be stuck there indefinitely.

▶ You no longer feel hesitant handing your wallet to salespeople and watching as they make change and return it to you.

▶ Throughout the course of the day, people ask, "Do you need some help with that?" in response to an ever increasing number of situations.

▶ Entering a number on a push-button telephone seems a never-ending challenge.

▶ You find yourself trying to get the best leverage to tear a check out of the checkbook.

▶ Hardback books feel as heavy as barbells, and the process of turning pages reminds you of pushing a rock uphill.

The list above is not the definitive list for all PD-surfers (this phrase sounds more adventuresome and life-giving than the phrase "sufferers"). I hope my descriptions made you aware of how it's an individual's daily choice how to deal with the many facets of PD. The fact that there *is* a choice makes dealing with PD easier for me.

IVAN SUZMAN, MAINE Since 1986, a time bomb has been ticking. It is likely to cause me great deterioration in the very near future. PD is so powerful that I often feel as if I am a marionette, whose strings are being pulled by an invisible, perverse choreographer....

I take four medications in an attempt to reverse paralysis. Without these medications, I cannot move. I am unsafe if unattended. My medications must be taken in varying combinations at 7:15 A.M., 9:30 A.M., 12:30 P.M., 3:15 P.M., 6:00 P.M., 9:15 P.M., 12:15 A.M., and 3:45 A.M. I never know with any certainty how well each of twenty-eight pills or partial pills will work. We PWPs all experience, eventually, this daily uncertainty.

Sometimes, the medicines hit me so hard that either I sway like the proverbial drunken sailor on a rainy pier, or they do not work, and I am stuck in a low-dopamine state of exhausting muscle pain, with knee and foot joints that arch as if to break my bones, and which will not straighten out and loosen up. My personal care worker is often busy with no letup for 3 hours, just to get me to the point of eating breakfast.

STAN HOUSTON A new neurologist about a month ago suggested I try a new combination of meds that seems to be working. Now, I'm "on" most of the day and evening and do not feel as time-constrained as when I could only count on 2 to 3 hours of "on" time in the mornings or afternoons. I'm getting a lot more accomplished most days. So now I don't feel so guilty during any "off" periods when I am forced to sit in front of the TV and wait until the next dose of meds kicks in.

Dyskinesia: A Common Side Effect of PD Meds

Dyskinesias are involuntary movements, such as fidgeting, wiggling, twisting, or jerking of various parts of the body, believed to be brought about by long-term use of levodopa medications. Dystonia, a drawing up or tightening of muscles, is another form of dyskinesia, often occurring in the feet and toes. These movements can range from mild sensations to disabling and painful and usually occur when one's levodopa dose is at its peak. Wearing-off dystonia, a drawing up or tightening of muscles due to falling dopamine levels, often occurring in the feet and toes, is a form of dyskinesia. Dyskinesia tends to be more common and more troublesome among young-onset patients than older PWPs.

NANCY MARTONE Unfortunately, after three to five years, the PD patient begins to experience some different symptoms caused by the medication. This is uncontrolled movement, called dyskinesia.

It may first show up as a head movement that can't be controlled. This is usually a "Yes"-type movement or a "No"-type movement. Personally, I prefer the "Yes" nod, although it is hard to say "NO" when your head keeps nodding "YES." I can't tell you how many refills on coffee or tea I've gotten when saying "no, thank you" while nodding "yes, please!".... Dyskinesia can get quite severe, with the whole body twisting and writhing in a most stressful way.[9]

SANDRA NORRIS When the Parkinsonian's body starts the transition from being "off" to dyskinesic, it is literally like a roller-coaster ride. The body goes through intense anxiety, heavy sweating, along with rapid heartbeats. Imagine Tina Turner doing "Proud Mary." The song starts extremely slow. By the end of the song…you understand what picture I am trying to paint. With dyskinesia the Parkinsonian does not have a choice or control of when or where these writhing body movements will begin or end.

DENNIS GREENE In my experience, mild- to medium-strength dyskinesia (not to mention many PD symptoms per se) can be reduced by a range of comfort-giving activities. These include emptying the bladder, putting on sunglasses on a bright day, taking off uncomfortable footwear, getting out of the heat in summer, getting into the warmth in winter, adding or removing clothing as required by temperature changes. *Nothing*, other than waiting it out, helps with strong dyskinesia.

LYNDA MCKENZIE, ONTARIO, CANADA Picture this: I decided that stucco would be an interesting effect on our bedroom wall. My innovative brain thinks, "Aha! Mediterranean effect, sun-washed walls, old plasterlike finish." No one else is home, but I am determined that this is going to happen. I find a giant box of pollyfilla in the basement and proceed to mix it in a big bucket. The fact that I want the walls to be pinkish prompts me to dump the pink paint into the pollyfilla; why paint it AFTER I've put it on, two steps in one makes a whole lot of sense to me. But I wasn't counting on quite THAT shade of pink....

So there I am, rubber gloves, giant bucket of too-pink stucco (I rationalize it will fade when dry), and four walls in need of help. Unfortunately, I feel the dreaded dyskinesia coming on, but looking at that giant bucket full of pollyfilla on the verge of solidifying makes up my mind for me. Onward!

Trowels, hands, all tools are brought into service. I like different effects. As I get excited about the wonderful results, the adrenaline kicks in and all limbs fly into noncoordinated action; bits of pink pollyfilla are being flung far and wide. I give up trying to wipe them off everywhere. I'll do that when I've finished.

Finally, I hear the garage door shut. Al is home. He comes upstairs to see what's going on. There, on the floor, scrubbing the globs of pink pollyfilla out of the gray carpet was the woman he married (so innocently, those few years ago), dressed in her birthday suit (everything else was covered in pink, crusty, rapidly drying pollyfilla), crawling around on the floor, knees a lovely shade of pink. Just another ordinary afternoon in the life of a PWP.

Living with PD: A Daily Heroic Act

According to Robin Elliott, executive director of the Parkinson's Disease Foundation (PDF), a 1998 study by the European Parkinson's Disease Association "spells out...with startling clarity what PWPs know from cruel experience—that living with the disease is a daily heroic act. It underscores the need for a worldwide commitment to uncover the cause of PD and chart its cure." Five thousand people in 11 European countries were questioned to assess the effect of PD on their daily lives. Some findings:

Tremor, poor balance, difficulty walking—at least 75 percent of respondents experienced these three common symptoms often or always in their daily lives:

- ▶ 80 percent had tremor.
- ▶ 75 percent had walking difficulty.

▶ 75 percent reported balance problems.

Fatigue from sleep disturbances:

▶ 93 percent said sleeping problems seriously affect their daily living.

▶ Almost 65 percent reported difficulty falling asleep.

▶ 75 percent found staying asleep difficult.

Depression:

▶ 80 percent reported feeling depressed or miserable.

Memory problems:

▶ 75 percent reported problems with memory.

Side effects of medication, such as dyskinesia or on/off:

▶ Almost 65 percent reported side effects from medications.

▶ 50 percent said side effects affected daily living.

▶ 67 percent reported wearing-off problems with their medications.[10]

MARY YOST, CALIFORNIA We're told that each person's experience with PD is remarkably unique. We're told that those of us with young-onset will live for many more years. (We're not told what the quality of that long life is likely to be.)

NANCY MARTONE For the most part, we're fighters, determined to keep as much of our mobility and abilities as we possibly can. We try not to be embarrassed by our peculiar posture, walk, strange movements and frozen facile expression—but sometimes we are.[11]

HILARY BLUE For myself, I am tired of having Parkinson's. I am tired of the continual encroachment on my life, on my usefulness, and on the time that is available to me to be a real person. I am wasting my day on longer and longer periods of dyskinesia alternating with bradykinesia and dystonia. I am requiring more and more help from others to keep up the appearances of normal living, thus '"wasting"' their life too, time they could be giving to a more deserving cause than helping me wash a few dishes, or just get dressed.

JERRY FINCH, TEXAS Many people have been diagnosed with PD and continue to live healthy, productive lives.

Mental attitude is half the battle in dealing with PD. There is no use in fighting the disease, but acceptance and determination keep many PD symptoms under acceptable control.

The other half is proper medication and information. If you are not receiving the correct information from a doctor—*change doctors.* Guilt, depression, anger are part of the acceptance process, and part of the healing. You will not die of PD. You can kill yourself with depression, but that is another problem. We have been given an extra reason to enjoy life, not to dread it.

Mo Udall

Morris Udall "let people know that he had the disease but said he didn't want to be a 'poster child' for Parkinson's."[12] He was determined to get on with his life and refused to allow the disease or people's reactions to it interfere with his work or his political aspirations. In spite of Mo's worsening physical condition, he delivered the keynote speech at the 1980 Democratic National Convention in New York City.

Eventually, though, the relentless disease made it difficult for Mo, a former star basketball player in college, to carry out even simple everyday activities—dressing himself, cutting his food, speaking, getting in and out of the car. His wife, Norma, recalled, "He never once said, 'Poor me.' He never acted embarrassed or depressed. He'd kid, when he couldn't get in the car, 'Look at me, Morris K. Udall, star athlete.'"[13]

The Losses Add Up

BARBARA PATTERSON, ONTARIO, CANADA Reading PIEN members' stories is both inspirational and heartbreaking. They say:

- ► I watch my body systems malfunction.
- ► I can't smell my food.
- ► My memory plays tricks on me.
- ► My hands can't do surgery any more.
- ► I fall asleep when I don't want to.

> ▶ My voice is weak and slurred, and my balance is poor.
> ▶ My gait is unsteady, and sometimes people think I'm drunk.
> ▶ My medication causes hallucinations and flashbacks.
> ▶ Too little medication, and lethargy drags me into sleepy oblivion; too much, and my mind races from thought to thought so quickly I can finish nothing.
> ▶ My wife has left for a life of peace and quiet, so I don't need to worry about the libido and impotence.

CELIA JONES, AUSTRALIA   I have since learned what he [my doctor] meant by "progressive." I used to associate the word "progressive" with something positive, forward-looking, innovative, favoring improvement. However, 10 years on, I can better understand what this word means to PWPs. Generally, as time passes, I am finding the medications becoming less and less effective and causing more side effects such as dyskinesia; rigidity and slowness of movement; loss of balance; digestive, cognitive and speech problems. The latter two problems were most responsible for my having to give up my teaching career early.

As I enter the advancing stages of the disease, I am often taken unawares by the insidious progress of the disease. It's frightening how valuable bits of myself—skills and abilities that I have always taken for granted—are being flayed off by the disease like bits of blown retread tires.[14]

Advancing PD

At end stage PD, patients may become completely disabled, helpless, and often confined to a wheelchair or bed. The following is Washington, D.C., journalist Mort Kondracke's account of Mo's last words and his final years with Parkinson's. Not every PWP will suffer the same fate, but it underscores the crucial need for fully funded, focused PD research, so that the recently diagnosed, and those already living with PD, will face a better future.

Udall announced after his reelection in 1990 that he wouldn't run again, but he did not make it to the end of the term. In January 1991, tired of watching an NFL play-off game, he decided to go upstairs to bed. "See ya later," he told Norma. The Udalls' Arlington townhouse has an elevator, but he hated to use it because if he leaned against the door, it would stop between floors, and he couldn't make it start. Besides, of all the afflictions of Parkinson's, the one he didn't seem to have was trouble climbing stairs. Norma says she heard him mount four or five steps. Then she heard him yell—and crash. She ran to find his head covered with blood. He suffered a concussion, four broken ribs and a broken collarbone and shoulder blade.

He spent weeks in intensive care at National Institutes of Health (NIH), then went to the National Rehabilitation Hospital. Then to the VA. He resigned from Congress in May 1991, two days after the 30th anniversary of his winning a special election for the seat his brother, Stewart, vacated to become John F. Kennedy's Secretary of the Interior.

"See ya later" were the last clear words anyone heard Mo utter.[15]

Udall spent the last 7 years of his life in a Washington, D.C., nursing home, unable to speak, swallow, or move.

Looking to the Future: Surgery, Research, Hope

KEES PAAP, THE NETHERLANDS/TEXAS The best meds for PD? Hope is one of the best, because it gives one a goal to live for. Our future might be the meds they are testing now. Research is not just important for finding the cure; it gives us mental support to keep on going, to believe in the future.

STAN HOUSTON Those of us who share this nightmarish neurological link often find our lives turned into a bad imitation of Lewis Carroll's Wonderland. Here, says the Mad Hatter, swallow this pill to stop those tremors. Sure, the White Rabbit chimes in, pop more drugs so your hands and legs will work. Say, the Jack of Spades muses as he waves his sword, how about a brain operation today?[16]

KEES PAAP Over the last few months, my PD has gotten worse and I am ready for surgery. I have been very overreactive, with wild days and much dyskinesia. Between those wild periods, I went "off" really bad, sometimes so fast that it seemed as if a switch had been turned. After 10 years of levodopa, the side effects are worse than the disease. My right arm sways in all directions and my leg joins the party.

It took me several months to get used to the idea of becoming a member of the "hole in the head club," longer than the one day it took to accept having PD at age 39. From that moment on, I tried to cope as well as possible. My quality of life had been good till the beginning of this year. Then it became worse, and finally it got bad enough to consider surgery.

(See Chapter 7 to find out what Kees decided.)

JUDITH RICHARDS, ONTARIO, CANADA As to the future, Al and I realize that things will get worse, but for now we don't dwell on what might happen. It's easier to take things day by day. There is a lot of research being done worldwide to help us manage better, and some of it may even lead to a cure.

I know two women who have had fetal cell implants. When I met one of them for the first time at a conference in Quebec City, she said she'd had the implant only 18 months earlier. She was up dancing, and she told me that before her surgery she couldn't walk to the end of her driveway.

I was asked a while ago if I thought a cure would be found in my lifetime. I thought for a moment before answering and then said, "Yes." We have choices. I have chosen to be hopeful.

(See Chapter 8 to learn about advances in Parkinson's research.)

These Companions/These Tears

BARBARA RAGER, ONTARIO, CANADA On the eve of celebrating my third year of membership in this weepy world of Parkinson's disease, I am learning to live with tears. They come when they choose. Empathy with a friend's sorrow makes them brim. A nearby burst of anger, a squealing brake, a ripple in a pond can bring them forth. I may be in a grocery line, or paused at a red light, when rivers of liquid grief flow over my shaking hands and soak my blouse.

This unbridled expression, this hot current of stormy tears is never liberating or stress relieving, as encouraging counselors promise. And if I do let go and really give myself over to the anguish, I'm there for awhile, sobbing and gasping for air, filling the house with a wrenched and twisting voice I cannot recognize as my own.

Unlike some of my fellow travelers on this road of chronic illness, I do not associate these outbursts with depression in the clinical sense. I've got a brain, which is degenerating at its own independent pace as I write and as you read this, in your home, or in the fidgeting quiet of a waiting room.

Does that depress me? Make me sad? Angry? Thrash about in despair? Yes. Even as I sense progress in the acceptance process, I continue to return from time to time to the torment of a dreaded future and to relive its desperate dance. I plunge into the well of self-pity and struggle with the destructive spirits that live down there. I unleash these terrors on my family, my friends, my colleagues, until they too cry out, "Stop!"

When I turn outward and allow the soft shell of healing friends to comfort me, I find it soothing. I also pursue alternative health paths, such as therapeutic massage, homeopathy, reiki.

These offerings from a far and distant time are empowering, regardless of their capacity to effect a "cure" as Western medicine would define it.

These tears are a part of this new coat I will wear for the rest of my life. Along with the slow freezing of my body, the letting go of my physical flexibility, my balance, my control in all physical functions and potentially some mental ones, the hurtful glances, the flaccid opinions of well-meaning people on how I should deal with my challenges, there will also be tears. Lots of them, more than I ever dreamed I could cry.

The tendency in our cinematic society is to finish this with an upbeat that reaffirms the gold at the end of the rainbow, to give the reader something he can take away with him, a reassurance in the basic goodness of life, or a renewed confidence in the effectiveness of a strong work ethic. Commercial publications want sales, and a heady, heart-throbbing ovation, with smiles and laughter, with tears being choked back by the sheer joy of the accomplishment in the face of annihilation—all this sells well. All I can offer, for now at least, is the tears. The story with a happy ending I'll tell another time.

c h a p t e r   3

Living with Parkinson's Disease I: Quality of Life

Journey to Wellness
BILL HARRINGTON

When diagnosed with Parkinson's
I vowed to fight it every inch
despite all I read
incurable, progressive
all the medical horror stories
doctors told me (for my own good)
even the atrocities I saw
inflicted on some victims

I stubbornly insisted
it would not conquer me
I would be the exception
not only that, this was my fight
and I didn't need any help
from anyone....

eight years later
the realization
I gravely underestimated it

I had fought exhausting battles
claiming occasional small victories
in an endless war, I could not win
instead of retreating, gradually, gracefully

I sallied forth on attack
a medical General Custer
surrounded outnumbered
increasingly humiliating defeats
my pride decimated

I cried out for help too late
the disease had a stronghold within me
a malevolent, cancer-like presence
it delighted in my despair
laughed at my tears
my bitter disappointments, its greatest triumphs
shrewd and calculating
cunningly persuasive
it turned my body against me
clouded my mind with morbid thoughts

arrogantly patient, knowing time was on its side
my pain gave it sadistic joy
it liked me to be afraid
of the all too real physical pain
but much worse
right from the start
this uninvited guest looked into my heart
to see what I dreaded the most
so it could make it happen
and discover what I loved best
so it could take it away

armed with that knowledge
it tortured me for years
I tried to reason with it
Threatened, cajoled, begged, bargained

but it is a formless darkness
driven by unreasoning hatred
it knows no mercy or pity

two years ago, it was nearly triumphant
I surrendered, tried to take my own life
I had no faith in myself or God
but He hadn't given up on me
He provided both a second chance
and the blessing of a new friend
who taught me that you only lose
when you give up
you never lose when you reach out to help others
if they turn away it is their loss
when you connect, you both win

armed with that knowledge
I started my journey back to wellness
I may never beat this terrible disease
but it can only make my life hell
if I let it.

Daily Life with Parkinson's

During a 1999 Senate Appropriations Subcommittee hearing, actor Michael J. Fox testified as "an expert (on) what it is like to be a young man, husband, and father with Parkinson's disease. With the help of daily medication and selective exertion, I can still perform my job, in my case in a very public arena. I can still help out with the daily tasks and rituals involved in home life. But I don't kid myself...that will change.... I can expect in my 40s to face challenges most wouldn't expect until their 70s or 80s—if ever."[1]

In addition to the daily medical difficulties in living with a chronic, degenerative illness, young-onset PWPs often face the compounded challenges of coping with jobs, children, spouses, and friends. They may face social isolation. Some live in poverty, brought on by forced early retirement and lost wages, denied disability claims and the loss of health insurance, as their medical expenses rise dramatically. Finding affordable assistance with daily living tasks can be especially problematic, if not impossible, for those on a limited income. Assisted living facilities for younger disabled people are rare anywhere in the world. Young-onset PWPs also face many more years of living with the uncertainties and progressing severity of the disease, and with the complications brought on by PD medications. In this chapter, we present a composite picture of "real life" with Parkinson's.

Changing Relationships

We want our friends to see behind our Parkinson's masks and beyond the physical changes our bodies undergo. We welcome their companionship and their understanding, but not their pity. Too often, it seems even old friends become uncomfortable around us or try to avoid us. We are still the same people inside.

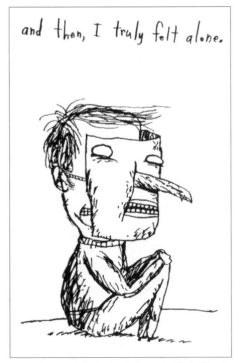

and then, I truly felt alone.

Maura Cluthe. *Behind the Parkinson's Mask: "I truly felt alone."*

RICK HERMANN, WASHINGTON Anybody out there having trouble keeping close to some of your old friends, now that you feature a progressive brain disease? I am noticing subtle effects, a kind of distancing, that I can't quite put my finger on. Part of it is that I'm just tired, and don't do as much as I did 2 years ago. I'm not feeling shunned, just a little ignored because I'm not out there socializing much. When I get done working for the day, I'm beat.

Old friends with good intentions send me articles about Parkinson's disease, but don't invite me out for coffee or to a movie. Weird.

DENNIS GREENE, AUSTRALIA Twelve years ago, I "came out" within weeks of being diagnosed. My family, friends, and acquaintances responded as individuals. Some, who for reasons of their own were unable to deal with the situation, dropped quickly out of view, never to be seen again; some were overwhelmed (and overwhelmed me) with pity, and these too, but this time by mutual consent, soon disappeared from my social circle.

But many of them accepted my new reality, made the necessary adjustments (and are still making them), and by so doing normalized my relationship to society as a whole. These people are the "gold dust at (our) feet," and the sooner we "come out," the sooner we can identify them and start concentrating on the relationships that are going to sustain us in the years ahead.

MARGARET TUCHMAN, NEW JERSEY Last week I was speaking with a friend, describing the various frustrations of PD: the unreasonable demands I put on myself; the erroneous attitude of not asking for—or allowing—help, while being disappointed that the unasked-for help is not forthcoming. These are the "head games" I play, and then I suffer the consequences. My friend asked me how often do I ask myself for help? How often do I offer loving and caring counsel to myself? If the roles were reversed, what suggestions would I make to a friend? Why do I feel that I am NOT WORTHY of the same consideration as I would give to any other human being?

JERRY FINCH, TEXAS

Dear Friend,

You haven't been by to see me in quite some time. I wondered about what happened, if I said something that offended you, so I started asking around. Word finally got back that you were uncomfortable around me because of the Parkinson's thing. That's why, instead of calling, I thought I might write you a note. Maybe I can explain a little better to you about the way I feel.

The last time you came over, I was having a lot of physical problems. Parkinson's is like that; good for 2 days, bad for 3. Before you come, call. I'll tell you honestly if I'm up or down. That way you know what to expect. But don't avoid me. Inside, I am still the same person I always was. I can still beat you at chess, still outtalk you over religion and politics. I can still laugh at all your jokes, still feel sad when we talk about some of our lost friends. I'm still me.

Don't be afraid to talk about the things you see. My hands shake; my walk is unsteady. I know that. It isn't a secret. I'll tell you about what I'm going through, about the medications and stuff. You need to know so you will feel comfortable when you see something happen. Parkinson's isn't contagious; it isn't even life threatening. Chances are, I'll live just as long as you, although I'm trying for one day longer, just to prove the point. Just because I've accepted having Parkinson's doesn't mean that I've accepted defeat. I'm still fighting. But the fighting would be so much easier if you were around. Why?

Because we used to talk about everything and I miss that. We used to laugh at stupid stuff and I miss that. We used to punch one another in the arm, work on our cars together, tell lies, talk about kids—and I miss all of that. We used to get sad together, remembering the things in the past. We made a vow never to talk about those things outside of our friendship and I need to talk about them with you.

I'm still the same. Nothing inside has changed, only the outside. That's why you don't need to feel uncomfortable around me. We've traveled too many miles together to let something like Parkinson's come between us.

So I'm asking you—call me. Come visit. Let's talk about today, tomorrow, 10 years from now, because the future will be so much richer if you're around, and so much poorer without you.

I might have Parkinson's, but you snore, so I'd say we're about even. I've missed you. As always, I'll be here for you, waiting for you to call.

Parkinson's in the Workplace

One of the first questions of many newly diagnosed PWPs is: "How long will I be able to work?" Of utmost importance in the minds of young-onset patients, this question at best can be answered with "It depends."

The nature and physical demands of one's job, the acceptance and support offered by employers and coworkers, the individual's response to medication, and the rate of the disease's progression all affect one's ability to continue working. Some PWPs continue to work for many years after diagnosis; others find that the physical and mental stresses of a full-time job become unbearable within a few years of diagnosis.

MARGE SWINDLER, KANSAS There are many, many issues that are peculiar to those who are still young enough to be working. As for whether to tell one's employer about the PD, it depends entirely on the employer.

If you work for a large corporation, you'll be on your way out the door as soon as they hear of the diagnosis. You may, have a job for several more years, but you'll no longer be seen as promotable or able to handle responsibility. I had friends we met through a PD support group who worked at the same corporation I did. They had chosen wisely, I think, not to tell our mutual employer.... I worked in human resources during part of my tenure for that company, so I know their fears were well founded.

On the other hand, the administrators at Dick's school system were very supportive and willing to do whatever he needed to prolong his teaching career. Dick has been on disability for 2½ years now, but managed to teach for 13 years following his diagnosis at age 37.

I also think it's fair, if you work for a small company, to tell your employer. They'll probably be much more willing to work with you than would a large corporation.

PHIL GESOTTI, VIRGINIA My decision to start medication immediately after diagnosis was based on the need to provide for my family and the realization that it doesn't get any better than this.... My neuro pointed out that I am in my peak earning years and I should make the best of them. The diagnosis has had positive effects. I leave work at a reasonable hour now. The management team recognizes that I can no longer physically work 60-hour weeks to help pull programs out of the fire. They happily take whatever overtime I can muster. I told my wife that if tremors eventually develop, or wild, uncontrolled movements, I'll simply move to Vegas and become an Elvis impersonator.

JEANETTE FUHR, MISSOURI As to employment issues, in my case, I had quit my tutoring job at our community college prior to diagnosis. My mom had been ill and I was not feeling well either. I might not have returned to work, but I had lunch with my ex-boss and she wanted to know if I'd like to come back. I explained I had Parkinson's and it was important that I keep stress low and I'd let her know. I then talked with my movement-disorder specialist about working.... I told him I missed the students. He said some PWPs like to and need to keep working, while others prefer quitting and having less stress in their lives. He emphasized that stress can increase the symptoms of Parkinson's.

I decided to return to work part-time. I also wanted to continue working in order to still be eligible for social security disability, which requires that a person be currently insured and have worked 5 of the last 10 years before permanent disability.

JANE BONANDER, CALIFORNIA Alan's occupation before and during most of his illness was systems operator for computer software. His last employer put a phone line into our home, so Alan worked at home for a couple of years before he had to retire because of his symptoms.

LINDA HERMAN, NEW YORK Before PD entered my life, preparing for a job interview involved updating my resume, researching the employer, and having my "interview suit" cleaned. Now with PD, preparation takes on a whole new meaning.

First, the big decision—to tell or not to tell. My first instinct is to be upfront about having PD. But realistically, if an employer has to choose between two equally qualified applicants, would they choose the healthy person or someone with an incurable, neurodegenerative disease? Legally, in the U.S., a job interviewer may not ask questions regarding an applicant's medical history, current illnesses, and medications; nor may they require a job applicant to take a medical exam. As long as a condition does not impact on the ability to perform the job, or require accommodations, I believe there is no reason to discuss it at the interview.

A job interview can be an extremely stressful experience, and stress can exacerbate PD symptoms. Some practical suggestions for surviving an interview:

▸ If given a choice, try to schedule the interview at a time when your medications are working at optimal effectiveness. It is usually not a good idea to suddenly change the established timing of your meds.

▸ Shuffling through papers can be difficult for tremoring hands, worse when one is nervous. Prepare a folder for each interviewer with your handouts or samples, and arrange any papers you will be using in strategic order.

▸ If your voice tends to become hoarse or strained, ask for a glass of water before the interview starts.

▸ Be aware of the Parkinson's mask. Make a conscious, extra effort to smile.

▸ Do whatever works for you to reduce stress before the interview—exercise, meditate, listen to music.

▸ Finally, study up on your interview and pre-employment rights under the law. Know what questions can and cannot be asked.

(Look in the resource guide (Appendix 2) for information on the Americans with Disabilities Act.)

RICK BARRETT, CALIFORNIA I'm a civil engineer who investigates disasters for a living. I work for a private company and as an engineering consultant. I regularly have to testify regarding my findings, and I am often involved in big money disputes—not the career path for someone with a thin skin or somebody who trembles.

I also am a member of one of FEMA's Urban Search and Rescue teams. I was in Oklahoma City following the bombing of the federal building. The end of my involvement with such things is in sight. I'm doing the best that I can. I like my work, and for some reason (maybe an adrenaline rush), when I am in the courtroom, my symptoms often disappear. On a couple of occasions when an attorney started questioning my body language, I've been forced to state as part of my testimony that I have PD, so please do not misinterpret my shaking and twitches for a lack of conviction regarding my opinions. This approach has worked well up to now.

In fact, my success in hiding my symptoms when I am at work has convinced many of my coworkers that there is nothing seriously wrong with me. I am currently cutting back on my hours and have filed for part-time disability. I know that many of my coworkers don't understand.

DIETMAR WESSEL, GERMANY I am 46 years old and have been suffering from PD for 12 years. The first 4 to 5 years were fine, without major problems. I could do my job (project manager for development aid projects in Northern Africa) without restrictions. My health situation deteriorated considerably from year 6 onwards. I had to give up my fieldwork and was transferred to another department. In 1999, I had to give up my job at the age of 44 and applied for and received early retirement.

I applied for the official status of a disabled person. Here in Germany, it means job security, since I can't get dismissed due to my disease. In addition, I can benefit from some special tax credits and other allowances. Is the social security for disabled persons similar in Canada and the U.S.? So far I have hardly met anyone working full time who's had PD for more than 5 years.

BARBARA PATTERSON, ONTARIO, CANADA I was diagnosed with Parkinson's in September 1992, and I am still working full-time, although it is becoming more difficult as Parkinson's progresses. I would like to be able to work until retirement age, but that is rapidly becoming an impossible dream.

JIM CORDY, PENNSYLVANIA I quit my job as a metallurgical manager in March 1995, when the stress and extreme fatigue proved too much. I felt like you feel after a Thanksgiving dinner—times ten.

JUDITH RICHARDS, ONTARIO, CANADA In the spring of 1996, I was forced to admit to myself that I could no longer do my job, and on the advice of the health-unit physician, I applied and was approved for disability. That was almost worse than getting the original diagnosis. It robbed me of my self-esteem and my self-confidence. And it began a year of hell.

DAVID BOOTS, CALIFORNIA It became increasingly harder for me to be as productive as my fellow employees. I worked with my union representative to write to my employers that "I am a disabled employee and wish to be accommodated in my job under the new ADA law." My employers did not accommodate me. They chose instead to document any and all shortcomings, and set up a system of harassment that was cruel.

After I threatened to file suit for discrimination and harassment, the city manager and the head of personnel quickly proposed that I leave immediately on long-term disability. So, at age 36, I retired on disability. This choice was definitely the best choice, since staying any longer would have produced stress that I was no longer capable of handling. However, they missed an opportunity to learn how to deal fairly and productively with someone with a degenerative neurological disease.[2]

(See the resource guide (Appendix 2) for information on the Americans with Disabilities Act.)

EMMA BENNION, UNITED KINGDOM I turned my anger and depression to constructive thinking, not destructive, and now work virtually full-time (as a volunteer) for the Parkinson's Disease Society of the UK and YAPP&Rs (Young Alert Parkinson's Partners and Relatives). It has helped me enormously, and although my family would like to see more of me, they appreciate that working hard for what I believe in is my way of coping with what the disease throws at me.

The Bottom Line: The Economic Costs of PD

The profound economic impact of PD on the health-care system and on the families of Parkinson's patients makes it "one of the most expensive neurological diseases treated on an outpatient basis."[3] The average annual cost of Parkinson's disease in the United States has been estimated at $25,000 per patient, including direct and indirect costs. Direct costs consist of expenditures for medications, doctors, hospital care, transportation, special equipment, and so on; indirect costs are those arising from decreased worker productivity and loss of earning ability, of both PWPs and their caregivers. The indirect costs are significant since so many younger PWPs are forced into early retirement.[4] As the baby-boom generation ages, the economic consequences of Parkinson's are projected to balloon. However, financial statistics alone cannot adequately portray the real costs to people's lives.

BARBARA MALLUT, CALIFORNIA I got my first, vague Parkinson's symptoms around age 32. And I'm meeting more and more PWPs who have had PD symptoms since they were in their 30s and 40s, "baby boomers" with long lives ahead of them.

Many of us live on limited incomes, derived from a variety of sources—Social Security Disability Insurance (SSDI) and Supplementary Security Income (SSI), decreasing savings, alimony, home refinancing. Often we must rely on caregiving and charity from family and friends. Along with our loss of financial and personal independence, our human dignity is slowly whittled away.

HILARY BLUE, SOUTH AFRICA/ISRAEL/VIRGINIA Our finances took a terrible turn for the worse, and we lost our house and ended up on welfare. Then my husband took ill—a very aggressive form of lung cancer (he was a heavy smoker). He was diagnosed and hospitalized on 8 December 1994. On Christmas Day, at 5 A.M., he died, 8 days after his 53rd birthday.

I was devastated. Here I was with three children, the eldest 13. Fortunately, Burt left an insurance policy, which allowed me to buy a house and a car and to put the rest in a trust for the children's education.

But otherwise, I had no source of income and no chance of getting a job. I had been tested a few months before by the department of vocational rehabilitation and found to be unemployable.

The little bit of money left over from buying the house and car was enough to knock me out of Medicaid, so now we had no medical insurance either. And we now had county social workers in our lives.

IVAN SUZMAN, MAINE I am a former medical anatomy professor. Now, with PD, I am dependent on donations of food for my pantry and freezer. With an income of $687 per month, which is derived from Social Security Disability Insurance (SSDI), and with a $708 per month Medicaid cap on total income, I am never able to produce enough income to live independently. My checkbook is frequently emptied before the 20th of the month. I know I could work part-time, but to pay my attendants, my doctors, and my prescriptions myself (without the benefit of Medicaid) would require that I amass $4,000 per month for these medical expenses!

RICK BARRETT My financial situation is changing in part due to the breakup of my marriage. I recently sold my house and am staying with friends while I look for a new place to live. With the divorce laws in California, I will end up splitting my paycheck—⅔ to my ex and ⅓ to me. I have no problem with paying child support, but paying an ex not to work does not seem fair.

My condition is such that I may end up on full-time disability within the next year or so. My company's long-term disability insurance only pays ⅔ of my original salary, and ⅔ of that will go to my ex. That leaves me about 22 percent of my current pay. It will be especially difficult after 2 years is over, when I will have to pay for my own medical insurance. I don't know what to do.

Disability Benefits in the United States

There are two forms of U.S. government disability benefits for those who are forced by medical conditions to stop working before retirement age. Social Security Disability Insurance (SSDI) is available for those who have worked and earned enough credits to qualify on their own work record. Benefits may also be payable to spouses, children, or survivors, under certain conditions. SSDI beneficiaries also receive Medicare coverage *after* receiving disability benefits for 24 months.

In addition, Supplemental Security Income (SSI) monthly payments are available for individuals who are over age 65, blind, or otherwise disabled, and who meet certain income and asset limits. Those who qualify for SSI immediately receive Medicaid coverage for doctors, hospitals, and medications.

For both programs, individuals must exhibit the specified symptoms of a medical condition that is recognized by the Social Security Administration (SSA). "Parkinsonian syndrome" is a recognized condition. In addition, individuals must meet the SSA's definition of "disability"—they must be unable to do work they could do before, or to adjust to other work, because of the medical condition(s), and the disability must be expected to last for at least a year, or to result in death.

It is recommended that applicants for disability make sure their doctors completely document all PD symptoms and any other related physical, emotional, or cognitive problems. Keep copies of all reports, correspondence, and communication. If your claim is denied and you wish to appeal, consider consulting an attorney. Some PWPs report that their claims were approved with no problems; others faced long, drawn-out battles with the SSA. (See the resource guide (Appendix 2) for suggested information sources on Social Security Disability.)

BARBARA MALLUT You have to understand that the words "positive" and "Social Security Disability" cannot be used together without the addition of another word, which is "lawyer." Now you have the magic key. It took me 3 years, the last two with an attorney on the job, to get SSDI after numerous appeals (and after having had PD for 15 years at that time).

CHARLIE MEYER, WISCONSIN I had no trouble getting Social Security Disability, and I didn't even want it, believe it or not. After I battled with my major disability carrier and had to hire an attorney to prove my partial disability just 2½ years ago and going on full disability about 1½ years ago, the insurance company last year insisted (and had the right to by contract) that I apply for Social Security benefits.

By being honest but not pushing, and certainly not exaggerating my symptoms, I was approved for benefits. I had another policy with a different company, and it also coordinated some of the benefits with Social Security. Therefore, getting Social Security I didn't want or need actually costs me several thousand dollars a year.

I am grateful to be in the position I am in, but couldn't Social Security have given the money to someone who needed it? This must fit under a corollary of Murphy's Law (or is it Parkinson's Law?).

HILARY BLUE Things began to go horribly wrong. My daughter Jessi's (age 9) behavior began to go out of control, and it was eventually decided by the various school and social-services people that she needed to be hospitalized in a long-term psychiatric facility. Maybe they were right; I don't know.

At the time I was vulnerable, and I was told if I signed her over to foster care, the county would take over all costs. If I had known better, I would have requested—demanded—help for myself, and refused to give up Jessi. I had no idea that I might be eligible myself for home-based care.

When I put in an application for SSDI based on my disability, including that list of reasons why I am unemployable, I suddenly learned that I am no longer eligible for Social Security bereavement benefits, which have been the cornerstone of my income since my husband died. Apparently, widow's benefits are only paid if you have in your custody a child under 16. Thus, when my children were put into foster care, I lost the right to collect Social Security benefits. Even though the youngest was 13 and back in my physical care, she was still legally in custody of the county, and even if I regain custody, I have lost the benefit forever.

So, when the county took my girls, they not only broke up my family, but they deprived me of my income as well.

An Unmet Need: Quality, Affordable Care for All PWPs

A survey on access to care for PWPs conducted by the Parkinson's Disease Foundation reported that only one in three respondents receive medical care from a Parkinson's or movement-disorders specialist. Only about 10 percent receive counseling or other social services. One-third of the respondents received no financial assistance for their costly medications. Long-term care—at home or in nursing homes—was rarely covered by insurance.[5] The most fortunate PWPs are blessed with partners who unselfishly provide care, often sacrificing their own lives and health. However, many PWPs are alone (sometimes as a consequence of being ill) and must somehow fend for themselves with little assistance available.

In 1997, Lonnie Ali gave this testimony at a Congressional Appropriations Committee hearing:

My experience as a Parkinson caregiver has given me greater understanding about this disease and how it can devastate not only its victims, but also family and friends as well.... I have had the opportunity to share my story as a caregiver with hundreds of others in Parkinson support groups. More importantly, they have had the opportunity to share with me their own personal stories of economic and emotional tragedy and hardship this terrible disease has brought them. In the course of our travels, I have met hundreds of Parkinson patients, some worse off than Muhammad and some not as affected. Muhammad and I have come away from these experiences with the resolve to help in any way we can to advance the research that will hasten the cure for Parkinson's disease.[6]

ALAN RICHARDS, ONTARIO, CANADA I have been asked what it's like to be a caregiver for a spouse with Parkinson's. I guess I'm qualified, because my wife, Judith, was diagnosed in 1993, and like everyone else with PD she had it for some time before the diagnosis.

So far the most difficult thing I've had to do as a caregiver is help Judith work through the stages of acceptance of her diagnosis. It was traumatic for her, as it must be for everyone who has to change a way of life, give up a career, and realize they will have to depend on others for much more than they ever did before.

But reassuring her that I'm in this for the long haul has helped, I think. And so has stepping back while she takes longer than she used to do many things.

Everything I've read about being a caregiver emphasizes that we need breaks too. We need to take care of our own health to be able to help our partners.

I know many Parkinsonians with physical problems, such as tremor and slow gait. I know their partners have different problems than I do, particularly with such things as helping with eating, or sitting up in bed, or lifting them up when they fall. Judith can do most of the things she always did. They just take longer.

All I have to do as a caregiver here is help with the housework, provide a shoulder to cry on sometimes, and hold the car door for her. I did all of these things before PD, to some degree, so life hasn't changed much. There's just more of it now.

For me, the best thing about my new job is that I can be helpful to someone who has helped me for many years. I can show my appreciation in tangible ways. I can be a care partner, not just a caregiver or caretaker. I kind of like it like this.

JOY GRAHAM, AUSTRALIA I am very conscious of the fact there are lots of PWPs without spouses to care *for* them as well as *about* them. What do we do if we're in that position?

RITA WEEKS, NEBRASKA One does not have to be single to have concerns about the lack of interest in treatment and care for PWPs. The problem seems a bit more prevalent with female PWPs than with male PWPs who are married (and I give my very sincere recognition of the support that some husbands offer in the care and support of their wives). Others of us wonder where the support will come from when we are no longer able to be in control of our days and searching for answers.

ANNE RUTHERFORD, NEWFOUNDLAND, CANADA PWPs who are able to live alone manage well until an unexpected problem crops up. This is not restricted to PWPs without partners. If, for example, our partner/caregiver must suddenly go into the hospital, where does the PWP go? What if family lives 1,000 miles away? Where I live, you get a respite bed in a nursing home—or a place on a waiting list!

HILARY BLUE We had to go through the formality of a court hearing. Imagine my horror when I got to the courthouse and found I was being charged with child abuse. *Child abuse!* Why?—because I had Parkinson's and was not able to give my child the care she needed. One of the "heinous crimes" I had committed was to do laundry by hand in the bathtub, because I didn't have the quarters to use at the laundromat.

Another dreadful "sin" was the children's ability, each one of them, to put a nutritious meal together. Jessi would probably have made a peanut butter sandwich with an apple and a glass of milk—but I was proud of my kids for that ability. The judge was horrified.

My legal-aid lawyer managed to get the charge reduced to "child in need of services," which I guess in a way was true. But what services?

If I had had help in the house, instead of spending hours taking care of simple daily tasks like washing dishes—a full day's job for bradykinesic me—when I wasn't shaking too hard to hold a plate without dropping it, I could have spent more time parenting.

SANDRA NORRIS, NORTH CAROLINA It is 3:11 early Tuesday morning and I am struggling with a few things. Struggling with the question in the back of my mind of just how much the PD has progressed...struggling whether I buy food today or I buy medicine today...struggling with my neuro about pain management. Being outraged over the unavailability of help for acquiring medicines.

No one should be faced with the question: Food today? Meds today? Family, do not get me wrong. I am blessed and thankful every day for what I do have. Yesterday I got word that I will have help with food. Still, drawing $736.00 a month in disability, when the cost of meds is $620.87, does not leave much to live on.

HILARY BLUE We were receiving medical care from a public clinic. A neurology resident from the local hospital came once a month for 4 hours. She saw everybody that had any sort of neurological condition and was swamped. Her way of dealing with me was to say if one levodopa doesn't work, take two, and if that is not enough, take three—and as my dyskinesia got worse, she told me to take more.

IVAN SUZMAN The central, unmet challenge that many PWPs like me face is our continuous vulnerability to institutionalization if we are single and either living on Social Security or low-income and lacking adequate support. How do we find adequate public or private caregiver funds?

My caregivers get paid by a Medicaid Waiver agreement between a payroll-writing company and the state government. We who are disabled are a small-budget group in the Bureau of Elder and Adult Services that has no remedy for younger, long-time disabled persons to receive care *at home*. It operates on a model that restricts us from full-time assistance at home and stops us from being truly independent.

I am now considered to be "nursing-home eligible," rather than given enough assistance to make a real stab at living independently and even contributing to the tax base. The personal-care attendants who assist me can come at the hours I choose, but the Medicaid Waiver program pays them $6.25 per hour. I therefore have an unstable workforce. At a fast-food restaurant three blocks from my house, the pay is $8.50 per hour and a medical insurance plan is available. My caregivers are not eligible for pay raises without an act of the state legislature. Some have not had a raise for 2 or 3 years.

CHRIS ROBIE, AUSTRALIA Here in Melbourne, Australia, our group of YPs (young Parkies) is suffering a crisis regarding our accommodation and care needs in the foreseeable future. Basically, our group of YPs has been diagnosed for 10 years plus, and all are under 60 years of age. In Australia, at least, there is very limited care and support for the YP, with most programs directed to aged people, and most do not take into account the special hardships that many young Parkies face.

The only real alternative offered by the government is nursing-home accommodation, where most of the occupants are very old, suffering dementia, and waiting to die. Not a nice place for an active YP.

The alternative is private care in retirement homes, hostels, or units, but they do not provide full-time care, and after the ravages of divorce settlements, many YPs have limited funds for the future. I might also add that after 10-plus years of PD, living on your own is a lonely and depressive existence.

It seems housing and care for young Parkies is a universal problem, and the problem is not going to go away!

What Can the Parkinson's Community Do?

The Parkinson's community needs to make a special effort to educate our elected officials, policy makers, medical personnel, and social services workers about the total impact of chronic disease on the quality of our lives. We need new models and paradigms for public health programs for PWPs and other disabled people. We need to develop pilot programs for younger disabled persons to receive care at home. We should appeal to our national PD organizations to provide leadership and funding to find solutions to the challenges of living with Parkinson's.

We believe that caring communities need to work together to find new ways to ease these burdens, not only for PWPs but for all disabled and chronically ill people. We offer a few ideas, proposals, pioneering programs, and dreams.

Helping Each Other

MARY YOST, CALIFORNIA   There's a stage for the PWP that I call the "sophomore years." We've made it past the trauma of the diagnosis, have realized that we're not going to become instant vegetables, and are trundling along okay. Severe on/off fluctuations haven't started, and we cling to the hope that somehow we'll never experience them.

The trick is trying to make sense of how best to use this time. We're needed to speak out, to raise funds, and to lend help to others—often those even younger than we are—who are in serious trouble. We also have to figure out how to best maintain our own health and to carry on with work and family obligations. Personally, "I'd rather burn out than rust out."

HILARY BLUE Do you remember a couple of months back when a plea was made on my behalf, asking list members to call a member of Congress from my home district, bringing to his attention my plight and asking for his assistance?

Well, it worked! I don't know who said what to whom, but yesterday, for the first of what I hope will be many times, a wonderful woman came to help me in my home. She is to come 12 hours a week and is to help me to do all those chores that have begun to be so tiring and so time-consuming for me. We spent a couple of hours just getting to know one another—she (hardly unexpectedly) had absolutely no concept of Parkinson's and how it affects people.

She is from Nigeria, and when she heard I am also from Africa, she jumped up and threw her arms around me in a big hug!

And best of all, she washed all the dishes in a flash and cut up a whole big pot full of vegetables so that I was able to make my kids their favorite stew for the first time in ages. Last night was a special one, for it is the first time in I can't remember how many months that we all slept under the same roof.

So to all of those who made those phone calls—you see, those calls did make a difference!

MARY YOST The PD village discussion was prompted by some of us who are solo, often because spouses understandably jumped ship after PD was diagnosed. There are enough of us that maybe we could become caregivers for each other. Every person has a dread—PD or no PD—of winding up in a nursing home, or worse, becoming a "burden" to our kids. Maybe that would be a solvable problem if we pooled our ideas.

CHRIS ROBIE Our Young Parkinson Housing Project is attempting to convince the government and support services that a specialized care and welfare program should be implemented. Justification for this special program is that the government will save considerable money if young Parkies are prevented from having to enter nursing homes—and there will also be a considerable decrease in the breaking up of families under stress.

Our initial dream of a Parkinson village comprising individual assisted-living units, hostel, and nursing home met with a lot of opposition, particularly from government and fellow Parkinson's sufferers. The fact that we had not considered at the start of the project is that Parkinson's sufferers diagnosed 5 to 7 years ago do not want to live with people who are further down the road, in the middle or later stages of the disease. This is pretty difficult to accept, but I think it's a fact of life. When you are first diagnosed, you tend to get on with your life and don't want to confront the issues that will ultimately cause a dramatic change in your life.

HILARY BLUE   One possible answer is the establishment of group homes—shared assisted-living facilities. They do not even have to be formal institutionalized arrangements. If several young PWPs set up house together, it would be beneficial to all concerned. The legal niceties would have to be worked out, but think of it. We all have different timetables for our offs and ons, so we would probably be able to assist each other through difficult times. And we would share caregivers, bringing down the cost and the number of caregivers, quite considerable for each PWP. And we would be of a similar age, and more compatible, than if we were thrown to the lions in a nursing home or similar institution.

Model Parkinson's Care Projects Around the World
Following are a few examples of model projects that demonstrate how cooperative efforts and some creative thinking can address the care needs of PWPs.

A Public-Health Program for Parkinson's
Quality, Access and Delivery of Parkinson's Care (QuADPaC) is a public-health research program of the Parkinson's Disease Foundation, initiated and directed by PIEN list member Dr. Perry Cohen. Among its goals are to "identify the unmet needs of the Parkinson's community...to build a foundation for delivery of comprehensive, quality Parkinson's disease care...to develop advocacy initiatives aimed at filling these needs," and to "facilitate the development of a 'National Parkinson's Care Action Plan' through the collaboration and support of a variety of public and private health organizations."[7] For more information, see the resource guide (Appendix 2).

Partnership Creates a Comprehensive Care Center

The Booth Gardner Parkinson's Care Center in Kirkland, Washington, opened in the summer of 2000. It was formed by a partnership of the Evergreen Hospital Medical Center and the Northwest Parkinson's Foundation, led by Bill Bell, another PIEN list member, and executive director of the foundation.

The center offers holistic, outcomes-based care, by a team that includes a movement-disorders specialist, occupational, physical, and speech therapists, a nutritionist, a counselor, and a neuropsychiatrist. Patients and their caregivers are consulted to develop a treatment plan that provides them with the highest quality of life.

According to Tony McCormick, manager of neurological services, "Besides helping patients and their families cope with the disease, the Booth Gardner Parkinson's Care Center is striving to educate the community about the illness and improve existing strategies for delivering care. I look at it as charting new territory."[8]

A Partnership for PWP Housing

Collaborative efforts in the United Kingdom between the John Grooms Housing Association, the Parkinson's Disease Society of the UK, Walsall Metropolitan Borough Council, and the Housing Corporation resulted in the Mali Jenkins House—a unique housing project for PWPs.

According to the John Grooms Housing Authority, "The project comprises 19 one-person flatlets, each with its own bathroom/wc and a small kitchenette. They are arranged in clusters with a number of small lounges around central communal facilities. The project aims to provide a sheltered environment for people with Parkinson's disease, so that they can live as independently as possible, while at the same time enjoying the care and security provided by a full-time warden and other support staff."[9]

Australian Support Group Tackles Housing Needs for Young Parkies

CHRIS ROBIE (APRIL 2001) When the Young Parkinson Housing Project started two years ago, we were optimistic of success. The past two years have seen us face a number of problems, and we have changed, modified, altered, upgraded, and downgraded our idea for care and accommodation for Parkies who are under 65 years of age.

We have developed an idea of "piggybacking" a YP section on an existing or proposed nursing home and have had meaningful discussions with a number of nursing home operators, who are also care providers. Of course they are interested in receiving a capital contribution for giving us bed rights, but it is far better to negotiate on this basis than to build and run a complete nursing home. Apart from the capital costs, the annual operating costs are huge and would deter most charitable groups. The fact is that Government support is necessary in building it and bearing the operating costs that are frightening, largely because of the labor costs of nursing patients. It has taken us 2 years to develop this piggyback idea, but if negotiations are successful, it will be the first specialized young Parkies section in a nursing home, with naming rights for our section of the building area, in Australia. It should be an example for other PD organizations.

We have also developed a house-sharing arrangement for young Parkies who are in need of some assistance but who are generally still operating in the community. This shared residence is overseen by a service provider who provides the essential services as they are required. There is a flexible written agreement among the occupants, but the success of the project relies on the compatibility of the occupants.

We believe the assisted shared-living arrangement solves the problem of loneliness, which we have identified as a major problem for young Parkies who are living on their own. I would stress that compatibility of the occupants is essential, and our trial house has a live-in caregiver who assists in the successful running of the house.

We are seeking funds from the government and philanthropic trusts to build further homes throughout the suburbs where the need exists. We hope that if there are a number of satellite assisted-living complexes, there will be a sharing and socializing among the various houses.

The success of our venture has been due to the adoption of our project by 300 businessmen/women who offer to help with community projects. They offered practical support, but more than that they opened doors that we would not have been able to get through on our own.

We have a long way to go, but at least we feel we are doing something about our future. Research is important, but you have to have care and accommodation to go on living and fighting. There is an urgent need amongst young Parkies around the world for care and accommodation. I would urge every YP support group to confront the problem. Don't put it in the "Too Hard" basket.

(See the resource guide—under "Parkinson's Organizations Worldwide"—for more information on the Young Parkinson Housing Project.)

Parkinson Village—A Fantasy

DAVID LANGRIDGE, UNITED KINGDOM Lying awake last night during the witching hour, my imagination began to run riot. Was there really a Parkinson village—a whole village inhabited only by Parkies—a sort of Parkinson's list in the flesh?

It would have to be in the depths of the English countryside. There would be lots of picturesque cottages with thatched roofs and roses growing over the walls; gardens full of hollyhocks, lupines, and foxgloves; neat little vegetable patches devoted to growing fava beans. Neighbors would greet each other with little remarks like "Come in and have some of my cider vinegar—it's very good for cramp." Or "There is a new man moved in to Honeysuckle Cottage—you wouldn't think he has Parkinson's— mind you, they say he is up to 3000 mg a day. He'll pay for it one day mark my words."

The village pub, aptly called the Parkinson Arms, would have a cheery "On Bar" and a more sedate "Off Bar." It would be noted for its Pub Grub, particularly its "All-day, protein-free breakfast" and its fava bean soup, naturally only to be eaten outside, weather permitting.

There would be frequent jollifications on the village green, including wheelchair racing and attempts to beat the record for the slowest 100-meter sprint. The village stocks would be revived and unhelpful neurologists pelted with rotten fruit. The village elders would discourage computers and Internet access to the listserv so that villagers would not be distracted from participating in the communal life.

Where, I mused, was this Parkinson paradise? Must be in middle England, not far from Stratford-upon-Avon, right on the tourist route, and might it attract flocks of visitors to view the curious inhabitants, just like the Amish settlements? Suddenly I began to think of the commercial possibilities and the opportunities to raise money for Parkinson research....

Life with Parkinson's Disease: A Terrible Beauty

DENNIS GREENE The progression of Parkinson's is so insidious that it is only in retrospect that you suddenly see, as Yeats put it, that your life has been "...changed, changed utterly" and that "a terrible beauty is born."

A terrible beauty. I don't suppose many here would take issue with "terrible" as an adjective for PD, but "beauty"? I must admit that there is nothing about the disease itself which I would describe as beautiful. But I have seen a great beauty in the way many in our community have risen to the challenge of living with PD. It's almost as if some people have a hard core, an inner diamond, that Parkinson's can only touch to polish. I have seen this inner strength in both PWPs and in caregivers, in the newly diagnosed and in "old-stagers."

It manifests itself as, among other things, humor, resilience, patience, humanity, empathy, concern for others, endurance, and determination. I believe that for those people who have this strength, it has as much influence on the shape of their lives, and the lives of those around them, as PD itself has, and underlying it, the one common ingredient—its foundation and also its driving force—is courage.

Now, I know, as do we all, that courage is not confined to the PD community, or even, indeed, to the world of the chronically

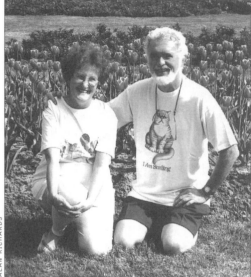

ALAN RICHARDS

Judith and Alan Richards visiting a "Parkinson's Tulip Bed of Hope," Rayner Gardens, London, Ontario

ill.... I also know that not everyone touched by PD responds courageously, but I, for one, have never before belonged to a community where courage is as widely spread or as readily shared as in our own community.

It is so "normal" amongst us that paradoxically it becomes almost invisible...and yet for me, moving in and being accepted by such company is one of the most profound and positive experiences of my life.

In 11 years of PD, I think I have heard discussion on just about every aspect of living with the disease. Every aspect, that is, except courage....

Acts of courage come in all shapes and sizes but most of them fall into one of two types. There's the meet it headlong—charge the guns...and then there is the War of Attrition type.... I think most people, should they ever think of courage in relation to PD, would immediately think of it in terms of the War of Attrition type, but I believe both types are well represented in our ranks, so I am going to look at charging the guns first.

Examples of courage under fire include:

▶ A newly diagnosed PWP and his or her caregiver simply coming to terms with their new reality.

▶ The same couple bravely fronting up to their first seminar or support-group meeting,...wondering how they are going to cope with meeting their possible future.

▶ PWPs and caregivers facing the milestone events, such as diagnosis, starting dedication, early retirement.

- Those moments when they realize that the PD symptoms have moved up a notch.
- Families making decisions about surgery.
- Going through surgery.
- PWPs and caregivers reaching out to help each other in support groups or individually.
- American PWPs ignoring their faltering feet and voices to lobby at the highest levels of their government for funds for PD research.
- Dealing with society's sometimes cruel judgments.

And then there is the other courage, the one that says, "hold on"; the one that hides itself so well because it comprises PWP doing the hard things, the things that take time and effort:

- The exercise sessions/the voice-training programs, knowing that they are fighting a rearguard action but unwilling to let PD walk all over them.
- Caregivers watching their loved ones suffer and keeping their concern hidden so as not to add to "their" Parkie's burden.
- Families making decisions about surgery.
- Again, a PWP going through surgery
- PWPs refusing to give in to the limitations imposed by the *ménage à trois* of tremor, rigidity, and bradykinesia, not to mention all their nasty little offspring. People getting on with their lives despite dystonia and dyskinesia....

And, last but not least, caregivers moving heaven and earth to help their Parkie live as full a life as possible, and somehow finding the time and means to live their own lives, too.

Tennyson wrote:

Tho' much is taken, much abides; and tho'
We are not now that strength which in old days
Moved earth and heaven; that which we are we are;
One equal temper of heroic hearts,
Made weak by time and fate, but strong in will
To strive, to seek, to find, and not to yield.[10]

chapter 4

Living with Parkinson's Disease II: Romance, Marriage, and Family

Another Country

BARBARA RAGER, ONTARIO, CANADA

"I was thinking," he says cautiously.

Oh, an original thought? My eyes fix on my lap. Perhaps a sports score? An "idea" for a room renovation he has seen in some restaurant? Maybe a retelling of a newspaper article, or what's his name's top-ten list for giving Pokemon to your boss. I'm all ears.

"It was a kind of thought, sort of a quiet thought."

My husband's body is bristling with sweat. He keeps lifting his T-shirt to his face to wipe his eyes. A vulgar locker-room habit.

"It came to me while I was mowing the lawn, a little while ago."

Now he thinks while mowing the lawn. I always thought he did it just to add to the stuff he could do without thinking, which kills most of his time, and which he can add to his own top-ten list of stuff he hates doing.

My right hand taps on the coffee table. It is not only from impatience. Parkinson's disease starts the right hand tapping from first consciousness in the morning each day. Now my left leg is going. God, will you spit it out. My heavy eyelids lift and land hard on his face. His eyes are averted. He is absorbed in a thing he is doing with his fingers on the back of the couch. We never look at each other any more. We sneak glances, then stray off. Afraid to see what, I don't know. After 25 years of marriage, there's not much we haven't seen of each other. Like now, his face draining of color, his fingers fidgeting. When did his hair go so gray?

"I was wondering..."

Get to the point. Please. Why can't we have a conversation any more? Everything out of his mouth lately has to go through this pause, hesitation, run it up the flagpole, send out feelers. Can't he just blurt it out?

"Well???"

"...if you loved me."

I corral my right hand, and hold it to tame the tremor that has suddenly become quite strong. It never used to be like this. Twenty-five years ago, we picked each other up on a 5-hour train ride from Ottawa to Toronto. Five hours of finding out that the one thing we both loved doing, the whole reason we had become teachers, lecturers, conference conveners, was because we loved to talk—to ourselves, anyone, and now each other.

I loved him immediately. It was his eyes, clear and ocean blue. His laugh always playing on the corners of his lips. The way he coughed into his pipe just after he sat down on the seat beside me, and then frantically tried to put out the sparks on his sweater with spit, making little fizzling sounds.

Five months later, barefoot on a beach on Prince Edward Island, at dusk, with a blessing from a minister once defrocked during the 1930s for his communist activities, with fishermen and farmers holding sunflowers, someone singing verse after verse of "The Ballad of the Flying Cloud"—another sunken-ship song—we took one another's hand and committed ourselves to each other and to life and love forever. A couple of flower children in jeans and cotton shirts, our own original ceremony—peace and love, a Volkswagen Beetle, macramé, and dreams: a long life, children, old age, bringing each other cups of tea in some future garden.

Our loving—once free and fun like tigers—has now, years later, faded into a shadow of halting advances and retreats. The anticipation of excitement and fulfillment is quickly replaced by the shame of being unworthy, spoiled goods, no longer eligible for the holiness of physical love.

Do I love you? Do I love you? How can you ask that? I'm gone. I've left for another country, a place for which neither you nor anyone else has a passport. A place that is entirely lonely, a place that separates me even from myself, where my body transforms daily into a stone, a shape with a purpose that is not mine. And where the best of all possible help comes from well-meaners in tones of, "Buck up, lovey, no one said this would be easy."

Our vows that day included an oath from the writings of Dag Hammarskjöld: Not to fail each other when the time comes to do the impossible. With the onset of Parkinson's disease, that time has come and we are indeed failing each other.

Have I not, several times, suggested divorce? That you would be happier with someone whole? That chronic illness kills marriages by the dozen? That if we separated, life would be just a whole lot easier for us both: fewer conflicts, fewer decisions to make, less need to conquer the gargoyles of intimacy that stand as gatekeepers whenever we attempt to touch the pleasure in each other, or the pain in ourselves. No longer would we stand naked before each other, and turn away from the memories of what was and our hopes for what might have been, had I not brought this monster in here to live with us. How can I receive your love in a heart that is fossilizing under layers of worthlessness and fear? How can you ask if I love you? It is you who cannot possibly love me.

The morning drips like an icicle into the afternoon. The quiet has not broken between us. He goes out to kill more time in the garden. I drift in and out of sleep on the couch. A dreamy, unhurried time. My hand tremor floats away as the stillness of sleep approaches. It is a trance: waking—tremoring; sleeping—at rest. Peace...

The door flies open and he's in the room. "I just got stung by a wasp. Can you see it? There, on my leg."

I arch my neck, oh yeah, wasp sting, too bad, does it hurt. Going back to sleep now. Within moments he's shouting, "Barb, my skin, it's on fire, I can't stop scratching. I'm swelling. Barb, my lip, look at my lip, it's swelling! We've got to get to a hospital. Barb, you've got to help me!"

We're in the car. His hands and feet, his mouth, steadily expanding. His eyes, his ocean-blue eyes, disappearing inside balloons of skin. Welts are rising on his arm. His breathing is becoming labored. My God. The traffic. The passage of happy aimless people driving lazily through a sunny afternoon.

"It's okay, honey, try to relax, think of something. Here, I'll put on the radio. Maybe a baseball game." Oh God, oh God. Slow down my tremor for the stick shift, let my leg work the clutch, please.

We're at the urgent-care clinic in eight minutes. He's seen and injected with adrenaline. We have to wait for the doctor to be sure the anaphylactic shock is over. We sit together in silence. I watch the redness of his skin fade, his eyes emerge as the swelling on his face recedes. His eyes blink in wonder and wide-open fear. His arms are folded tightly across his chest, as if holding his life together. One shudder and he'll fly apart.

We are alone in the waiting room. I move closer to him and curl my arm around his shoulder. His breathing softens. In this still, throbbing moment I remember the time when we arrived home after the final diagnosis which confirmed that I had Parkinson's disease. Clinging together here, in the stark awareness of our sudden frailty, I think of how he took me by the hand, led me to the couch, and folded me in his arms. Hours passed as the afternoon light faded away and the room engulfed us in darkness. The still, silent presence of his body, the closeness of his breath, the calming rhythm of his heart confirmed for me then, as mine confirms for him now, that we will be there for each other forever, and beyond forever.

Love Comes to Call: A Conversation

LYNDA MCKENZIE, ONTARIO, CANADA When I was diagnosed, my life was full. Making a living and raising my kids took most of my time, but I did miss "the male influence," so I tried to fill that void. I went to dances, read the personals (and answered a few), got sent on some memorable blind dates, and even joined a dating agency—lots of fun but nothing serious.

I could tell there were no possible serious relationships because I told none of my dates about my Parkinson's. I was still able to conceal it most of the time, and if they noticed a tremor, I replied quickly that I was shivering, or nervous. Stiffness was sore muscles from an overzealous workout the day before. I was a master of disguise, and my excuses worked every time. But then, in August of 1992, I went on a blind date. Al was different.

KEES PAAP, THE NETHERLANDS/TEXAS I'm very pleased to inform you about a big change in the life of two of your list members. The first list member is Faye Armstrong, and the second one is me. Faye is a general surgeon and became a member of this list because a friend of hers has Parkinson's. We met when she was on holiday in Holland, and we fell in love. So much in love—we call it "love at first sight"—that we can't live without each other.

BARB MALLUT, CALIFORNIA "Real life" means that once you meet someone with whom there's a mutual "chemistry," see each other enough times, and do enough things together to build a mutual history, you get to the place where you have a "relationship."

There's a point when the reality of being with an individual who has a chronic disease begins to seep through.

LYNDA MCKENZIE I had to tell Al right away about my Parkinson's because I didn't want him getting interested without knowing there was a lot more to me than met the eye. I was also protecting myself. I didn't want to depend on him and then find out that he didn't know if he could handle it. So, after trying to figure out a good way to introduce the subject, then realizing that no way is a good way, I blurted out "I have Parkinson's." He was driving at the time. Al pulled over to the shoulder, stopped the car, turned towards me, took my hand, and said, "Well, I have no idea really what that involves but I have a feeling I'm going to learn."

KEES PAAP I told Faye about my PD, and she knows exactly what it is, but her answer was that health is not important if one loves somebody, even if a severe disease such as PD is involved. Yesterday she said to me (when I was very off), "I love you, Kees Paap, whether you have PD or not, are on or off, because inside you is the man I love." I love Faye very much and I want to be with her day and night. So I asked her to marry me and she said yes.

FAYE ARMSTRONG PAAP, TEXAS From the recently single and not-with-PD standpoint, I can say that a problem like PD will certainly make you take a good look at the person inside and out before you decide to marry him. Probably, more people should do that before they marry anyhow. But if you see someone who is worth having, then you will want them regardless of a disease. How do any of us know that we will have years of health? We could be hit by a car or struck by lightning at any moment.

BARB MALLUT There's also the family and friends of the "well partner" working on them out of concern that they might end up saddling themselves with a person who's potentially going to be severely handicapped. That is not something the family takes lightly.

FAYE ARMSTRONG PAAP Many of my friends and family asked me why I would marry Kees knowing that we faced a strong probability of hard times in the not so distant future. My answer was always a question back to them: "If you had known at the time you got married that your mate would be in an accident and be paralyzed in 10 years, would you still have married him/her?"

The answer was always preceded by an expression of surprised understanding, then: "Of course! I would not have given up the good times."

LYNDA MCKENZIE PD really isn't an issue on its own; it just happens to be a part of me. And now that we've made that lifelong commitment, it's a part of him too. Silly of me to have worried that he wouldn't be able to handle it.

We were together constantly that fall, engaged in November and married the following June. I knew I could live with this man who took Parkinson's in his stride and who accepted it as just another facet of me.

BARB MALLUT I'd like to point out to my fellow Parkies that at one time those of us who vowed to "Love, honor, and cherish, in sickness and in health," probably knew next to nothing ourselves about Parkinson's disease, or any other major chronic disease. And we'd never even heard the word "caregiver" in relation to a spouse or life partner, much less figured we'd end up in that not always enviable position.

ALAN BONANDER, CALIFORNIA If we could look into the future and see what were to happen, including sickness and death, I doubt any of us would get married, have children, or want any long-term relationship. Interestingly, about a month ago, a member of my support group—someone with PD—got married. His wife-to-be had visited our group and asked what she would be getting into by marrying someone with PD. We were not very supportive of the idea. No guarantees in life.

A Wedding Invitation to 1,700 Online Friends

13 February 1998

Dear list friends,

We can't send everyone an invitation by snail mail, that's why we're doing it this way:

> *Kees asked Faye to marry him, and she said "Yes!"*
> *Since then, their love has grown deeper, so*
> *He will ask her again on*
> *Saturday, February 21, 1998*
> *Faye Armstrong and Kees Paap*
> *together with her parents*
> *Mr. and Mrs. Ralph W. Armstrong*
> *Invite you to join them to hear the answer*
> *and celebrate their wedding.*

Learning to Live with a New Marriage Partner

Dr. Michael Rezak, medical director of the American Parkinson Disease Association (APDA) Young Onset Parkinson's Information & Referral Center states, "Special attention must be paid to the effects of PD on the family. In the young-onset group, individuals are just beginning families, and children are of school age. This is the time of life when family activities begin and financial growth occurs. The stress of dealing with a chronic disease is difficult and can take its toll on intrafamilial relationships. Added to this is the frequent accompaniment of depression, anxiety, and sexual dysfunction resulting in a chaotic situation that often requires counseling in order to preserve the family unit."[1]

LYNDA MCKENZIE We really had no role models; all the other couples in our group had Parkinson's invade their lives after they had already been together. It was something they hadn't bargained on, even though they'd promised in sickness and in health. I know for many of our friends Parkinson's has thrown a twist into their lives that has not been easy to deal with. Almost-overnight role reversals try the most stable relationships.

STAN HOUSTON, TEXAS I seem to be busier now as a disabled retiree than when I was a working stiff. (Forgive me for that obtuse pun.) I am the housekeeper/business manager/bill payer/grocery shopper/cook for our country home in Cat Spring, and there's always something my wife Shirley wants me to do.

Example: while she was getting ready for work this morning, I had to protect her from a baby mouse that wandered into our bedroom. Picture this: PWP in pajamas, robe, and slippers, with NO meds in him—clinging to a walker with one hand and brandishing a fly swatter with the other while yelling, "Get off the bed and chase him over here so I can hit him!"

AUTHORS' NOTE: Stan Houston died 3 June 1998, from complications of Parkinson's.

JUDITH RICHARDS, ONTARIO, CANADA Being a perfectionist and always extremely independent, I now felt worthless. I couldn't do anything right. I tired easily (and still do) and couldn't keep up with my housework and gardening. I felt guilty because Al was doing things that I should have been doing, and at times I felt I had ruined our lives. I never went through the "Why me?" or denial stages, but I was angry and frustrated—mostly with myself for any number of reasons. But Al bore the brunt of it because he was there. It began to affect our marriage, to the extent that Al and I were referred to a psychiatrist. We both needed counseling. I had become a different person, and Al didn't understand why or how to deal with it.

RICK BARRETT, CALIFORNIA I've been a member of this list for a few months now and have found it to be very helpful in dealing with the issues surrounding PD. My wife of 8 years, on the other hand, has been wrestling with my diagnosis without the help of any support. She has expressed to me her interest in corresponding with others in her situation. Unfortunately, she doesn't want to be on anyone's "list" (caregiver list). We are in our mid-30s and have an 18-month-old son. I was diagnosed with PD about 4 years ago.

New Pathways to Communication

In addition to affecting movement, Parkinson's disease is also a disorder of communication—diminishing body language, facial expression, and speech. Often we unconsciously hide our emotions behind the Parkinson's mask, creating barriers between us and those we are closest to. Others may remark that we have sad or angry expressions, which discourages inter-action. Our voices lose expression and volume, and we may find ourselves unheard or ignored. We need to discover new ways of sharing our emotions and ideas with others, and they need to become sensitized to our communication difficulties.

JOHN QVIST, SWEDEN I wonder: where do we set the limits as to what we tell our loved ones, girlfriends, boyfriends, wives, husbands, best friends, family? Should we always share everything, or is that cruel? Should we always hide what isn't obvious about our grief and illness?

I, of course, understand that the answer isn't simple.

Speaking for myself, at first I felt that saying everything was just too much. I could not put that load on my wonderful girl-friend, who already worried enough about my health.

On the other hand, I always asked her to accompany me to my neuro, so that she could ask questions. In that respect I didn't dream of hiding the facts from her. It was just my fears for the future that I mostly kept to myself. "In sickness and health, for richer or for poorer..." How does it go?

Now, a few years later, I feel that keeping your partner out of your feelings is not right—not to mention the fact that it is very hard to hide feelings from someone you're living with.

MARGE SWINDLER, KANSAS If you don't tell your friends and children, that makes your spouse your only support group, and that's a horrible position to put one in. My husband did that for something like 12 years, and as his condition progressed, it became increasingly difficult for us both. I might add that about the time he was diagnosed, the same symptoms that led him to see a doctor in the first place became noticeable to others. How-ever, he had created such a wall of silence around himself and the subject that none of his friends or family had the temerity to approach him directly. They asked me instead. We ended up with this little conspiracy of silence, which did none of us any good.

JO GREENE, AUSTRALIA In 1987, Dennis was diagnosed with Parkinson's disease, and his body language slowly faded in front of my eyes. That animated face, his easy smile and wave, his being relaxed or tired, content or anxious, looks that I knew so well, things that I could read easily about him with a quick glance or longer gaze were gone. There was many a time I would think that he didn't like something because the emotion wasn't there for me to see. In fact, the emotion was there, but he just couldn't show it.

His emotions are on the inside—locked in by the Parkin-son's, unable to be seen because of the rigidity, slowness, and masked expression. This, in a man who is full of sensitivity and tenderness with such feeling for the world and the written word. It's frustrating sometimes for me not to get immediate feedback. They say patience is a virtue, but for Parkies' partners, it's a necessity to keep the very important channel of communication open. I'm still working on it. The Parkinson's won't go away, and the "channel" gets slowly more blocked.

So, we have to find other ways to get messages from our partners. Talking is of the essence. We must not be afraid to say what we feel to our partners or fear hurting their feelings a little bit—they have a right to know.

RICK BARRETT As my disease progressed, my wife's ability to deal with the issues at hand became less and less. She didn't understand the on/off phenomenon. When my face went blank with a Parkinson's mask, she would get upset and demand that I smile.

RITA WEEKS, NEBRASKA I just read that a caregiver had said, "My husband can smile when he wants to," and I must add two cents from the PWP here. You are right, the masking is a part of Parkinson's. You err in "can smile when he wants to." I recall the first time I saw a video of myself walking. I had always assumed that if I held my head up and smiled while I was struggling, no one would notice that I walked a little different. The video showed not only a problem with gait, but I was not holding my head up and smiling—this came as quite a surprise to me! My husband will frequently comment on my expression as being a bit sullen, when I thought I was smiling. Smiles come from deep inside. For some of us, they don't always show on the surface.

JOAN SNYDER, ILLINOIS I didn't realize that my mask was so noticeable, until my kids (eight and ten) asked me why I was never happy anymore. They were hurt that their homemade Christmas gifts weren't the huge hit that they usually were. Since then, I have made a real effort to speak more with my eyes. It has been a hard thing to accomplish and takes a real effort on my part. It never works when I'm really tired, but I think it's worth the effort to really be there for my family. I didn't believe that it could really work until I told my husband that I loved him and he said that he knew—he could see it in my eyes....

Now every so often, I will see glimpses of startling maturity and gentle, little kindness in the midst of their youthful frenetic energy. Oftentimes a kiss must take the place of a smile that won't show on my frozen face—sometimes it must be a frozen claw on an arm, demanding that they look into my eyes to see how much I love them.[2]

Weathering Changes and Crises in Marriages

JERRY FINCH, TEXAS   There is no doubt that the physical problems associated with PD affect virtually every facet of our lives. We lose our jobs, we stop driving cars, former friends drift away, and if we are lucky, new friends come. It would be unreasonable to expect it not to have a major influence on our marriage. The balance of shared responsibility, of equality in duties, becomes a thing of the past as we enter into the phase of caregiver/patient. Slowly the duties of marriage, of day-to-day living, become more the responsibility of the caregiver, as the patient becomes unable to do the things once done with ease.

RITA WEEKS   I cannot speak for the single PWP, but if there is a married couple on this list that can come forward and tell me that the marriage has not been grossly changed by their Parkinson's diagnosis (or prediagnosis), I would like to hear their story. Somehow, I think what I would more likely hear is how the "crisis" has passed and perhaps how things have changed since they have weathered that time.

ALAN RICHARDS, ONTARIO, CANADA   I know my experience has been unique. So has every other caregiver's. It is said that Parkinson's is a "designer disease," and no two people have the same symptoms or problems. That's true also for the caregivers, partly because of the differences between patients, but also because of personalities and habits and many other factors.

Some couples have gone through hell in their relationships since diagnosis. Others have been able to carry on with their normal lives, making minor adjustments to accommodate changes as they appear. Judi and I have been somewhere in the middle.

BARB MALLUT I believe as awful as this disease is for us, it's just as awful for our spouses and life partners. It's just a different kind of awful for them. It takes a very special partner to hang in there for the long haul, and a very special relationship.

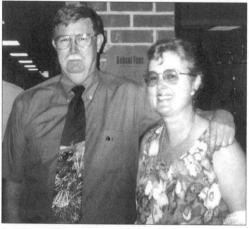

Jeanette and Leo Fuhr

JEANETTE FUHR, MISSOURI My marriage partner of nearly 27 years has been my rock this last couple of years. When we said, "Until death do us part" at ages 20 and 24, we never knew how stressful a diagnosis of a chronic illness could be. Thanks to my husband's patient, determined notion that we can survive my Parkinson's, I have transformed from a stunned, sobbing, depressed female to a roaring woman with Parkinson's. Of course, I give myself some of the credit. My list family, my own family and friends, my neuro, and my God all said, "It may not be easy, but we'll get on with life."

BARBARA BLAKE-KREBS, KANSAS My husband, Fred, took the diagnosis in stride. Ever since we fell in love in 1981, he has let me know day after day, by both word and deed, that he loves and respects me, as I do him. As much as possible, we allow the other independence and support in pursuing career and community-service endeavors. Over the years, we have adapted in a variety of ways to my current abilities (his too—after all, we are all getting older) and have tried not to let PD limitations disable us from pursuing dreams and opportunities.

For example, in 1996, Fred became a district governor for Rotary. Normally, the DG's spouse accompanies the governor on visits to clubs. As this would have been too strenuous for me, Fred asked me to write a column for the DG's monthly newsletter instead; it was very well received. To make up for not getting out very much socially, we try to have friends over here. (Have I mentioned that Fred loves to cook? Also, we rely on take-out quite a lot.) Life is an adventure, and PD is a part of ours.

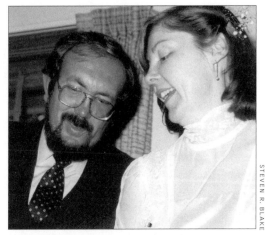

Barbara Blake-Krebs and Fred Krebs at their wedding (October 1982)

STEVEN R. BLAKE

LINDA HERMAN, NEW YORK On the day I received my diagnosis, my husband, Ed, told me, "Our future might be different from what we thought it would be, but we will always have a future and I will always be there for you." He's repeated this many times since. He seems to sense when my thoughts about the disease's progressing overwhelm me and how much I need to hear those words over and over again.

DONNA TESTA, NEW YORK That old saying stands out in my mind: "Until you walk in my shoes, you have no idea what I am going though." I wish I could go back over the 27 years I have been a nurse and have carelessly said to my patients, "I understand what you're going though."

Five years ago, my husband and I were sitting in front of a nervous neurologist, who as kindly as possible said four words that changed our lives forever: "John has Parkinson's disease." The right-hand tremor that had brought us searching for answers was given a name finally. Since that time, there have been many visits to the neurologist and many symptoms such as the blank "mask face" and an increase in tremors. There has also been a continual changing of medications and dosages to keep up with the endless progression of the disease. We always have had a close relationship, but fighting this disease has brought us even closer. We appreciate each other even more and live each moment to the fullest, knowing well that no one has any guarantees in this world.

MARGE SWINDLER Mr. Parkinson has taken up residence in my home, uninvited, and made my life and my husband's much more difficult. It has taken a toll on our patience, our family life, and our pocketbook.

There are times I can sit back and think about how fortunate we are to have medical help and to live comfortably, with all the modern conveniences. I can also appreciate the fact that Dick is doing exceptionally well for someone who has had PD for 18 years. I do admire his determination to hang in there and not let PD stop him, no matter how difficult some things are for him. Nevertheless, I have to do things, or learn to do things, that wouldn't be expected in the normal course of events. I'm all too human, and there are times when I'm simply seeing the half-empty glass and feeling the anger and frustration of dealing with the day-to-day losses and difficulties PD has brought into our lives.

RICK BARRETT I'm certain that my difficulties in dealing with the disease played no small part in my wife's decision to divorce me to look for something better. We saw a counselor for a while, whose main experience with PD was dealing with older patients in the final stage of life at hospices. I get uncontrollable spells of tears when I am at home. I worry about the future. My first neuro indicated I would have about 5 years before the progression of the disease would become disabling. And even though my present neuro disagrees with this prognosis, I often am pessimistic, perhaps due to seeing my own grandmother struggle with the same disease until her death this year.

NANCY MARTONE, TEXAS As the symptoms progress we tend to socialize less and less. While part of this stems from embarrassment, it also comes from the fact that the areas of the brain that are stimulated during social events worsen the PD symptoms. So, a fun time isn't fun anymore. It's a real chore. This too causes stress in the family. Communication is of the essence![3]

ALAN BONANDER There have been too many times when I have put PD ahead of my marriage. We are prone to assume that our care partner/spouse will always be there. Marriage needs work all the time.

AUTHORS' NOTE: Alan Bonander died from complications of asthma in August 1996. His wife, Jane, sent the following message to the PIEN list in response to the many heartfelt tributes to Alan:

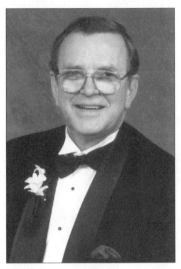

Alan Bonander

JANE BONANDER, CALIFORNIA
Thank you, all of you, for your wonderful words about my husband. We celebrated our 33rd wedding anniversary in June 1996, and I wanted to share with you a part of Alan that you probably didn't know. He was "the son of a preacher-man." His father, both grandparents, and other relatives, on and on back into history, were ministers and missionaries. But Alan marched to a different drummer, no matter how many times his mother urged, in her subtle way, that he follow in the footsteps of his ancestors.

His analytical mind was ripe for the computer age, and he was a genius at it. Then along came Parkinson's—that nasty, greedy disease that began to rob him of his strength, his desire to work with his hands, his outer self. Because of his interest in his disease, he became the minister, the missionary his parents had wanted him to be. I have no doubt about this, especially when I read all of your comments. Sharing what he knew gave him pleasure.

I will admit that many times I cursed the computer age, for he spent hours and hours and hours on the Internet, sharing, advising, helping, while I wondered if he would ever take a few minutes out for himself. The thing was, he was doing this for himself. It made him feel good.

He was a great husband and father. Brother and son-in-law. My parents couldn't have loved him more if he were their own. And he was a missionary extraordinaire.

Sexuality and Parkinson's Disease

LYNDA MCKENZIE Parkinson's has a way of reducing things to
the basics. One of the most important basic needs is intimacy,
emotional and physical. Maybe things have to be different from
the way they once were, but that's okay. We can compensate,
adjust, and improve with just a bit of effort in order to retain
the ability to bare our souls and bodies, allowing ourselves to be
intimate with another human being.

When my body feels rigid and nonresponsive, when each
movement is difficult, I don't feel at all attractive. When something as simple as a smile is so difficult, it's easy to perceive of
myself as undesirable. Those are the times when the only reason
I want to get even close to a bed is so I can pull the sheets up
and hide under the covers.

But having a partner who realizes my frustrations and doesn't
dwell on them makes those feelings easier to deal with. Silent
reassurance, cuddling, and no expectations help reassure me that
he still finds me desirable. To know that the person I love wants
me, no matter what, goes a long way towards helping me deal
with my unresponsive and plodding body.

I often feel as though I do all the taking and my partner does
all the giving. It's difficult to take an active part in lovemaking
when arms and hands refuse to move. But patient gentle caressing
and whispered words somehow get through my limbs, touch my
core, and make me feel wanted. I feel sexy and loved when I am
with my partner. I feel normal. How wonderful that is!

JERRY FINCH Being a male, I can only relate this from a mas-
culine point of view. I would think that females feel a parallel
sense of loss, a deep change in the sense of sexuality. The
essence of manhood, the self-assured acceptance in the world of
football and cars and Saturday-afternoon lawn mowing, of having a few beers with the guys, of hunting and fishing and hanging around the hardware store fade into history as the new
world of medications, stumbling walks, and shaking hands
moves in as a replacement.

Within the relationship of marriage, the essence of sexuality
also changes. The questions arise in us of our mate's desire
within the scope of our physical appearance. Of course, we are

the same person, but love and desire sometimes take separate paths. The concept we hold of ourselves becomes different; feelings of self-worth, of acceptance, become clouded by our disability.

This is when love must change. It must become wider than before, more willing to accept the faults, the failures, and the physical appearances. Either accept or fade away, to become just another memory. Lovemaking comes either from the desires of closeness, caring, and a deep bond of love or from a desperate attempt to regain a lost past. As often as we try to rise above the physical, we are reminded that we are physical. We cannot deny our existence—physically, spiritually, or sexually. To do so is to admit defeat to our disability, to give up a part of our lives, to let part of ourselves die.

I am blessed to have a caregiver who shares with me the strength of love that allows us to see sexuality beyond the physical. On the porch at sunset, watching the pastels of the day give way to the stars of night, or at three in the morning when I scream out in pain from a combination of leg cramps and twisted muscles and tremors, she is there, holding and caring, willing to accept me for what I am. When our desires lead to caresses and nowhere else, I know our love is deep enough to find satisfaction in a gentle touch.

When it comes to surveys and statistics, I think it really doesn't matter. That I don't have 2.3 orgasms per week, or 3.4 attempts, is not what my life is all about. At this point in my life, sex and love are the same; they are held together in the eyes of my wife, in a smile, in a soft and warm kiss.

How many times have we made love? Once. It began the moment we met, and will not end until both of us take our last breath.[4]

PD and Kids

As list member Rick Hermann points out, parenting books don't often include advice on telling children about Parkinson's disease. There are few how-to guides written for parents about coping with chronic illness while also keeping up with the physical demands of active toddlers or weathering the emotional ups and downs of typical teenagers. Sharing experiences, problems, and ideas with other parents with Parkinson's can be invaluable—even if the other parent is an ocean away.

Susan Reese, Coordinator of the APDA Young Parkinson's Information and Referral Center, advises:

Parkinson's disease is a family affair. Children will raise questions and concerns related to having a family member with Parkinson's disease: "Is it contagious? Is my parent going to die? Was it caused by something I did? Will it get better?"

The lack of facial expression exhibited by most Parkinson's patients makes children wonder if their parent is continually angry or sad. Children need to be reassured and to have their questions answered directly and honestly. Older children require concrete information about the disease as well as emotional support.[5]

JEANA BARTLETT, GEORGIA There are more and more of us young ones out there. Funny, we consider ourselves "old" when we are in our 40s, but in PD that is very young! Children need to understand what the effects of PD are. I made the mistake of not involving my boys too much…just didn't talk about it. It needs to be a family affair.

RICK BARRETT We've had two children—a daughter, 1, and a son, 4. This year there has been a lot of critical illness among grandparents, so he equates tremors and frailty with a "grandpa" and loses sight of the fact that I am his father.

RICK HERMANN, WASHINGTON Yesterday I gave my 12-year-old son the news that I had Parkinson's disease. I had been thinking for a while about what to say, whether to say anything to him directly, as he has asked me in recent weeks about my shaking hand.

"Will your whole body start to shake?" he asked. Tough question! I told him I was taking good medications that really help me keep symptoms minimized and that I'd be okay for a really long time. "But does it get worse as time goes on?" he persisted. "Yes," I said. "But it's going to happen very slowly." We talked a little bit more, until he seemed okay for the time being, and later I asked Lee if she thought I had done okay. "I thought so," she said, "but he's really worried about disease."

He is. But the truth is, Eli has two really good parents who will continue to take care of him and nurture his budding independence as he moves into his teenage years—and believe me those challenges have already begun. I feel like we'll be okay in the larger picture, and we try to pass that outlook on without minimizing his fears. It'll come up again, I'm sure. This isn't in any of the parenting books that I've read!

IDA KAMPHUIS, THE NETHERLANDS   Twelve years ago I was diagnosed with PD. I have a son and a daughter who are now 24 and 22 years.... They were too young to be able to understand what was happening to me when the illness started. My son's reaction was the easiest for me. He was helpful when asked. He was not indifferent but did not talk, and not knowing whether he wished to was the only difficult thing for me.

My daughter was very angry with me. She did not want to hear anything that referred to my illness. She was embarrassed seeing the embarrassment of others, but at the same time felt very guilty about her own reactions. I tried to tell her that her anger was quite normal, and that I too felt angry sometimes. An example of both of our angry reactions occurred when we went to town together to buy some clothes. She got angry because I was dyskinetic. I, angry too, gave her a train ticket and said, Go on your own. Act as if you don't know me and go home. After such rows, I felt guilty and I feared she would grow up avoiding anyone with a disability who reminded her of the pain and anger she felt about her own mother. My wish to do something to prevent that was in conflict with my wish to protect her against sorrow at the moment.

After some time the problem moved to the background. We all got rather used to the situation, and the children were growing up. We had a reasonably good life. For the children, bringing friends home was not a problem. They told every new friend about my disease. I never noticed any of them being embarrassed. The weekend evenings in our house were a coming together with the friends of both our children.

I now make a jump in time. My son started his university study. He came home from his first week at school and told us about a student in a wheelchair. My son had talked quite naturally to this boy. However, to his surprise he was the only one who could do so. He had realized he owed this to his experience with me. So, I had my turn to be surprised....

My daughter went to the university too. Coming home on weekends, it was difficult for her to see me off. My symptoms were increasing, and she saw it clearly. She said she could not bear to see me suffering. At that moment it seemed to me not wise to protect her by hiding the symptoms. I told her my disease is very serious indeed and of course, it is not easy, but that I was alive and I valued life. I told her some people think having a disease like PD makes one live in hell. However, she could see for herself that this was not true, and she did not help me by making my suffering her suffering. *Things like that need much repetition.* It is okay for our children to enjoy their lives and we need to tell that to them. The moment finally came when she read a book about biological psychology and read about Parkinson's disease. She started asking me questions. A few weeks ago she said that she felt more grown up than some of her fellow students because of what had happened to me....

Reading stories like mine are useful even if you do not agree with my ideas for how to talk to our children. Thinking about your own opinion is easier when a contrasting opinion is available. We need to think about how our disease affects our children and our parenting, and how to talk about it with them.[6]

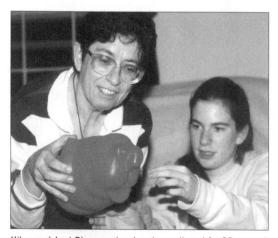

Hilary and Jessi Blue counting donations collected for PD research

HILARY BLUE, SOUTH AFRICA/ ISRAEL/ VIRGINIA I have just received a letter from my lawyer. In it he states, "It will be very difficult to have a plan other than permanent foster care approved given the timeframe in which

Jessica has been in a return-to-home plan." In other words, our time has run out.

She has been in limbo for too long. She is in an after-school program that is only available to kids in foster care. Nobody can explain why this is so; it would make far more sense if she went to school from my house in the morning, then to this program, and then came home in the evening. But to be in compliance with one regulation or another she has to stay in a foster home.

And she is only allowed to see me every other weekend. Thank heavens for small mercies—this has just been extended to the whole weekend.

So what can I do but breathe a deep sigh of regret and resignation and thank all those who have helped me fight and learn to accept that my daughter's teenage years will be spent with somebody else's mother...except for every other weekend.

Describe the Pain: Stanza Three

RITA WEEKS

Did you know I was in love with another person too?
Did you know that I loved Superwoman?
I chased after her for years.
She was there so he could be in the lab and still be Dad.
She was there for the Brownies, Cub Scouts, and just kids.
She could rustle up dinner for 12 or dessert for two.
Her windows and floors sparkled.
She had time to listen.
She wore high heels and Pendleton plaids and chased a
*   title.*
She was one of our best workers, always an extra mile
*   (or smile).*
She disappeared without a note, no wave good-bye, no
*   fond farewell.*
She left both of us searching for the one we loved.
Does it hurt? Describe the pain.
Would you ask again, if I did complain?

"May I Have This Dance?"

DAVID BOOTS, CALIFORNIA He strode confidently into the
party catching the eyes of several women in the room. He felt
great at the moment, the medication was working just right for
a night of fun and frolic. He was "on" and several people
stopped and told him how good he looked. Chris just beamed
and thanked them in a warm, even voice. He made his way to
the open bar in the far corner just as someone tapped him on
the shoulder.

"Chris?"

He turned around and saw his old girlfriend, Ann O'Reksia.
"Ann, how have you been?" he said (noting how she still
seemed too skinny).

"Good gosh, Chris, you sure look like you're doing better
these days," she gushed.

Chris Kinesia hesitated briefly before answering. It's true that
his medicinal intake had finally become regulated and also
included vitamins and homeopathic additions. But attitude and
determination had also played major roles in this change as well.
He resolved never to give up hope that someone would find a
cure in his lifetime.

"Thanks," he replied. "I'm watching what I eat and try to
exercise some each day."

He continued, "Are you and...?"

"No, we gave up on trying to make things work. Hey, can
we talk about something else?"

"Sure," he said, "Would you like to dance?"

Ann extended her hand and he led her on to the dance
floor. They moved from memory as the music took them back in
time when everything had seemed a lot more simple. She felt
wonderful in his arms, and during the slow dances she held him
close as his cheek caressed her hair. He didn't want this night to
end and told her so. She responded by holding him even tighter
as the music played.

"Chris, you don't realize how hard it was for me to break
up with you. I don't know if it was the PD causing you to lash
out at me and others close to you but it scared me. And now,
you remind me of the Chris I fell in love with years ago: warm,

self-assured, and friendly. Tell me this is real, tell me that we can work things out this time."

"Ann, I still have PD but it's basically under control now. I've done a lot of work on my health and my attitude and feel I have emerged a better person for my efforts. When I was in the middle of it, I was too self-absorbed and angry at life to contemplate the number of people I was pushing away from me. Now, I'm ready to start again. If you'll take me back."

She reached up and pulled his face close for a kiss. He responded by picking her up and spinning her around while never breaking the kiss. It was a moment right out of the movies....

"Chris," his caregiver called from downstairs, "we're gonna be late for your neuro appointment. Do you need some help getting ready?"

"Will you just give me a friggin' second! I'm getting there," he yelled back as he sat twisting and grimacing on the edge of his hospital bed, his socks half way on his feet, his shirt and pants hanging on a nearby chair mocking his efforts. He knew that eventually the caregiver would come to dress him and dry his tears.

He knocked over his plastic drinking cup, spilling juice all over himself. He began to sob. He only had dreams and memories of how things used to be. His arms flailed about as he tried to direct his muscles to cooperate. His caregiver, hearing the commotion from downstairs, took a deep breath, and entered the room. "You're just having a difficult time right now, Chris," he said as he helped him to his feet.

Trying to be lighthearted, he asked Chris, "May I have this dance?" This time, it was a long while before he could stop crying.[7]

chapter 5

Invisible People:
How the Public Perceives
Parkinson's Disease

Eyes
BILL HARRINGTON

*I feel the weight of their eyes
watching me, my strange contortions
I look up angrily to challenge their gaze
they glance away
I drop my eyes like unexploded bombs
please, not this again!*

*my arms and legs dance to a primitive rhythm
I can't hear or control
I abandon my body to its fate
and retreat deep inside myself...
why do I bother going out?
do I have a masochistic ego?*

*inevitably Parkinson's symptoms ambush me
intensely private battles*

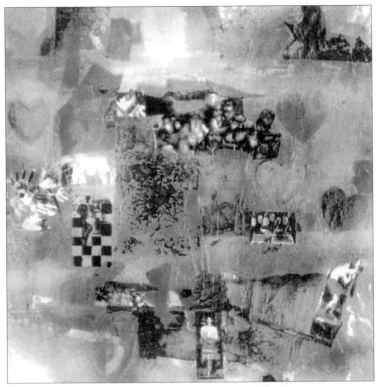

Lillian Duck. *Eyes.* Mixed media (acrylic on canvas, tissue paper, magazine images, gloss). Exhibited with poem by Bill Harrington in Vancouver, B.C. (1994).

in a public goldfish bowl
escalating in duration and intensity
have left me frustrated, humiliated
vowing bitterly not to leave our home's sanctuary
gradually, I regain control
but this skirmish leaves my mood
in blackened, smoking ruins...

For now, as close to "normal" as I get
this is just a temporary interlude
my pendulum has already begun its journey
to the other dreaded extreme
that equally unpleasant time

of rigid, awkward movements
like the flawed puppet of a demented master
muscles tensed like clenched teeth
in uncompromising spasm
PAIN, vanquished briefly
returns with a vengeance
to reclaim its bitterly relinquished throne
as king of the Parkinson's symptoms

ironically, from the recent uncontrollable movements
it is a remarkably short trip
to being barely or unable to move at all
my body stops contradicting my brain's commands/pleas
instead chooses to ignore them completely
these periods of terrifying complete immobility
are aptly termed freezing
time seems frozen as well
captured inside a stone statue
in a park filled with pigeons

I know if I have taken my medication
it is a matter of waiting for it to work
but when you are out in public
seized up like an unlubricated tin man
with back spasms so severe it is hard to breathe
minutes seem like hours
I get desperate, will take anything
just to move again
so I often take extra medication
which causes horrible cramps
in my legs and feet
hobbling is barely possible with assistance
of my wife and/or my faithful cane (Able)

Eventually the cramps are replaced by
the period of extra movements
the cycle complete…
So it is far better, easier

to go home now
during the calm time
in the eye of a hurricane
while I can leave
with some vestige of dignity
once there I take refuge in my room
and suffer in bitter solitude
away from prying, spying
eyes.

Perceptions and Misperceptions

Tremor is...people looking at your hand instead of
listening to your ideas. MARVIN GILES

Visibility stands for the extent that people see you as the
person you are in spite of the symptoms. IDA KAMPHUIS

Are people with Parkinson's really invisible? To the general public—who know little about the disease, and even less about its
occurrence in young people—in a sense, we are. To those individuals who choose not to look at or to see others who are
physically disabled, disfigured, or just different, PWP are indeed
invisible. Health-care providers who do not recognize the
unique problems and needs of younger Parkinson's patients do
not see us as we really are.

Parkies may add to their invisibility by hiding their symptoms out of fear or shame. Faced with an uncompassionate
society, we often build walls to shield ourselves from hurt and
rejection. Finally, advancing PD severely limits the ability to
interact and communicate with others, resulting in an ever-
deepening withdrawal from one's community. Slowly but surely,
Parkinson's victims fade from the public's view and attention,
and do become invisible to the world.

A 1997 study conducted by the Pacific Parkinson's Research
Institute found that while the existence of Parkinson's disease

is widely known, the severity of the condition is completely underestimated. Although 94 percent of the respondents had heard of Parkinson's, and at least almost all respondents could describe some of its characteristics, fewer than 10 percent of the respondents could describe the totality of the effect that Parkinson's has on an individual.[1]

Two years later, it was reported that "although more people have Parkinson's than multiple sclerosis, Lou Gehrig's disease and muscular dystrophy combined, the disease has escaped much public notice and research funding."[2]

Parkinson's disease expert Dr. Erwin Montgomery acknowledges, "Little is known about the unique effects Parkinson's disease has on younger people. Most of the medical textbooks have been written based on experience with elderly patients. It has only recently come to light that significant numbers of young people develop Parkinson's disease. As health care professionals we need the young patients to educate us, so we can understand what they are facing."[3]

Describe the Pain: Stanza Four
RITA WEEKS

You have no tremor, aren't you lucky
Someday soon they'll find a cure.
The news is full of wonderful stories
I saw a man dance down the hall,
St. John's Wort and blue green algae
will help you if you start to fall.
At the health store, hear their story
Don't trust your doctor for goodness sake.
You have no tremor. You are not twisting,
But you do look tired, do you lay awake?
Does it hurt? Describe the pain.
Would you ask again, if I did complain?

IVAN SUZMAN, MAINE Parkinson's has been projected as an old-person's terminal disease, creating a stereotype that is completely inappropriate.

CELIA JONES, AUSTRALIA Certainly, in Australia, Parkinson's disease has mostly been associated with the aged and has been portrayed by the media as inflicting a "mere hindrance, a bit of a tremor." When my neurologist told me that I had Parkinson's 11 years ago and asked me what I knew about it, all I could think of was that it was a trembling that usually occurred in very old people. There were hardly any books available, and most of those only dealt superficially with younger-onset victims.

If I tell anyone I have PD, they either don't believe me, as they don't associate Parkinson's with anyone under 60, become overly solicitous, as if I've told them I have terminal illness, or, much less frequently, ask me to explain what it is.

DAVID BOOTS, CALIFORNIA I'm constantly amazed at people's varied reactions to my situation. A coworker once told me, "David, if I were in your position, I'd probably be mad." To which I replied, "Yeah, but then what?" Others have told me, "David, I just want you to know that I think you're very brave going through this." To which I replied, "What's the other choice?"

LYNDA MCKENZIE, ONTARIO, CANADA It is amazing about the PD awareness in our own families, isn't it? I know my parents didn't realize for the longest time what dyskinesia is and how it works. They had seen milder cases, but when I had a good session at dinner a few months back, they didn't know where to look.

DENNIS GREENE, AUSTRALIA I have never been so proud of my daughters as the day, at ages 16 and 9, when they stood beside their grossly dyskinetic father and "stared down" a huge crowd of high school students who had actually formed a ring to gawk.

DONNA TESTA, NEW YORK Dealing with the public is always interesting when you have Parkinson's disease. Unless people are familiar with the many different symptoms of the disease, such as tremors, rigidity, and "stone face," they react in many different ways. But through it all, people with PD and their loved ones learn to deal with the many situations that come up and sometimes even find some humor.

My husband, John, needed a new car. Realizing that the usual bargaining that goes on with buying a car is stressful for him and brings about increased tremors, I decided to try and start the bargaining over the phone with the salesman, explaining why. He had not had any experience with the disease, but assured me that if we came down he would deal with us in an honest manner. I meanwhile set about reassuring my husband not to worry, as I had researched everything, and all he had to do was sit by while I finalized the deal.

At the car dealership, we went through the usual introductions and were taken into the salesman's office. He seemed to forget what we talked about over the phone; as soon as we sat down, he started the usual wheeling and dealing. John jumped up and said, "Let's go!"—his face rigid and his tremors going a mile a minute. I turned to the salesman, who looked scared and about to cry, and I said bluntly that he had lost our sale. He spent the next five minutes apologizing to us, and turned things around with a good offer. We decided to take the offer after I spent the next 15 minutes educating him about PD!

Where is the humor in all this? Maybe it was because the salesman really was sincere, or maybe it was just to get rid of me after my 15-minute lecture, but for the first time in my life, I knew we really got a fair deal buying a car!!!

Becoming Invisible

As symptoms progress, everyday participation in society becomes more difficult for PWPs, and gradually we fade from the public's view and awareness. Testifying at a 1998 Congressional hearing on Parkinson's research funding, Joan Samuelson, founder of the Parkinson's Action Network (PAN), explained how PWPs become invisible:

Every person afflicted with Parkinson's can describe the effort to manage their medication so they are at their best when out of the house. And then, one day, that person starts disappearing, as the act of coping becomes too much. Perhaps if we died soon as a function of Parkinson's, its impact would appear more dramatic. Instead, we slip out of the func- tioning world and are forgotten.

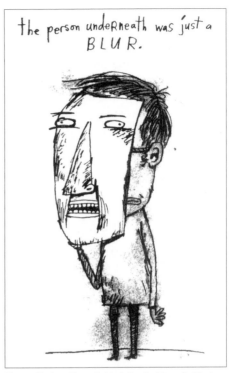

the person underneath was just a BLUR.

Maura Cluthe. *From Behind the Parkinson's Mask:* *"the person underneath was just a blur."*

The impact on our visibility...we start out courageously trying to power through our dis- ability, ignoring it, even hiding it, to maintain our normal lives. We end up silenced and impris- oned in our homes, our care facilities. In either case, there is an insidious ingredient: our suffering has been rendered invisible to the outside world.[4]

JIM SLATTERY, AUSTRALIA I have discovered another aspect of PD—invisibility! As PWPs, we are invisible to some of the populace. I had long suspected this, as at meetings, dinners, etc., I would talk, and no one would hear me, or I would stand up, wave, dance on one leg, or do whatever was necessary to attract attention, and no one could see me.

The real proof came when, because of a heat wave over Christmas (here in the land of Oz, it is frequently in excess of 40 degrees C—105 degrees F—over the holidays), I shaved off my beard and mustache of 20 years standing, and *no one noticed!*

I was mainly out with my wife, helpmate, and primary care- giver. I think people noticed me as a sort of Jim-shaped blob appended to her and figured I must be her husband. This occurred even with close friends.

Seriously, I think people with disabilities, particularly those disabilities that make others embarrassed or remind them of their own human frailty, are seen "out of focus," if at all.

If, added to that, they have difficulties in communicating, e.g., shaky handwriting, slurred speech, etc., they are further shoved to the periphery of people's minds.

How "visible" are PWPs to caregivers of long standing, to relatives, friends? I have made it one of my New Year's resolutions to REALLY see and hear ALL people, not just the more visible ones. (Now, I wonder how invisible I am in the bank?...)

JO GREENE, AUSTRALIA

Dear Jim:

It was amazing that your post came through a matter of hours after we had been discussing the very same thing. It had occurred to me for some time, months, maybe longer, that people just don't "see" Den. They see him but don't really SEE him. Your description of a "Jim-shaped blob" is sadly accurate but very true. Den doesn't have to shave off a beard not to be noticed by some people—he just stands there and isn't seen, or worse, is seen but not acknowledged as a thinking, functioning, human being.

That very day you wrote I ran into someone whom I hadn't seen for awhile. Den was right at my shoulder—just standing. She fixed a gaze on me and conversed, actively avoiding any eye contact with Den (whom she knew). I wondered when she was going to ask him how he was...but it never happened. I must confess that it bothered me, but Den said, "Well, that's how some people are." I said, "Why must it be?"

Some friends of ours (he has Parks) went into a shop for a watch. He asked what they had (he was dyskinetic), and the shop assistant then asked *the wife*, "What sort of watch would he like?" "Not one from this shop anyway," he said, and they left!

I know in my heart of hearts that it is the other person's problem; they are uncomfortable, uneasy, etc., but I don't feel any better, and I don't suppose other sufferers/caregivers do either. You have touched a spot here. Thank you. What is sad is that everybody has something to offer, but their disability may prevent some from being "read" as they rightly should be.

(Oh yes, good luck at the bank!!!)

JOY GRAHAM, AUSTRALIA My husband is badly affected by speech problems—out of proportion to the rest of his problems. He walks and moves quite well and never shuffles, so he is not immediately obviously "disabled." In restaurants I have found that if he is not understood, I am immediately questioned—usually by eye contact—to explain on his behalf. We have a sort of unwritten agreement that if the person is not in a tremendous hurry or is the sort who is happy to wait until Bob tries again, I hang back with my mouth shut.

Another aspect of "invisibility" that happens to many caregivers is when a friend will go over the top (almost) in asking about the PWP—either directly or indirectly—and will NEVER ask, "And how are YOU doing, Joy?"

IDA KAMPHUIS, THE NETHERLANDS My equilibrium is disturbed, and it happens that I fall and need help to stand up again. When that happened in my own neighborhood, I learned just how much people I don't know at all do know me, and know exactly where I live. So it seems my visibility is not lower but higher than that of others. But this is visibility of another kind.

It happened once that I was in town (in The Hague) and I was going "off" and could not walk anymore. I entered the most nearby shop, explained in a few words what was going on, and asked to call a taxi. This situation brought about the same helpful reaction.

More difficult were situations in which I traveled by train and became dyskinetic, a situation in which other people are confronted with me, without being expected to do something. In situations like that there is much embarrassment, and other people made me feel as if I had some highly contagious and disgusting disease. I also experienced this same reaction in other public places like supermarkets. People often stare at me but immediately turn away when I look back, and they startle when I come too close.

HILARY BLUE, SOUTH AFRICA/ISRAEL/VIRGINIA I tend to stay at home, except for an exercise class for those with advanced stages of PD. One of the reasons I can't go out is that I physically cannot get to places. I can't drive anymore, and I am dependent on other people to take me out. Sometimes it's just easier to stay home and have food brought in, than to go out and have people looking at me as I drop my food all over the place.

Describe the Pain: Stanza Five

RITA WEEKS

Window shopping is all you're doing?
How about lunch at the new cafe?
So I park the car and shuffle over
Will I walk a block or two?
Who will stare and who will ponder
what is this strange dance I do?
Will I dribble, choke, or stutter?
Will I freeze or shake today?
Will you listen while I wonder
just how to cope from day to day?
Does it hurt? Describe the pain.
Would you ask again, if I did complain?

Building Walls

The frozen expression of the Parkinson's mask adds to the invisibility of PWPs by preventing our true emotions from being revealed to others. Additionally, PWPs often construct psychological walls to protect themselves from society's probing eyes and expected rejection. If built too high, though, these walls also fortify the layers of social isolation between PWPs and their communities.

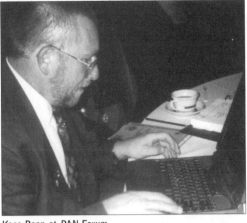

ART HIRSCH

Kees Paap at PAN Forum

KEES PAAP, THE NETHERLANDS/TEXAS I have a lovely daughter, who is in high school. She is 18 years old and studying psychology and social communication. She gave a personal presentation about how SHE thought that I protect myself against the world, including my family. She built with big wooden blocks a wall between me (played by herself) and the outside world, and next to each line in her paper she placed an arrow, ➤, as a mark for pushing a block away from the wall, in this way tearing down the wall.

Here is the text of her paper; my daughter wrote as if she were me:

The Wall

This wall I built against the community, to keep my disease behind and to protect me and my surroundings.

Block 1: This block I use to keep up appearances against my relatives and especially my family.
➤ But this is not necessary because they want me as I am.
Block 2: This block is necessary for my concentration. As a symptom of my disease, it is hard for me to concentrate, and because of this I am soon chagrined.
➤ When I have to concentrate, I can say so and don't need the block.
Block 3: With this block I prevent my feelings from being hurt.
➤ By being open, I can prevent being hurt.
Block 4: This block is built from the frustrations that I can't do certain things anymore, such as writing and playing the trumpet.

➤ But there are many other things I can do, like playing volleyball.

Block 5: This block is a symbol of my medicine, which prevents me from getting a good sleep.

➤ But I can fill this time by doing things I want to do.

Block 6: This block is for my disappointment that I can't do my job.

➤ But I do have the opportunity to lose myself in computers.

Block 7: This block is built from the many accumulating activities I want to do for the society.

➤ Many positive things are part of this, such as beautiful journeys.

Block 8: This block stands for the difficulties I had accepting my disease.

➤ But fortunately, I had much help.

A Father's Response

The wall exists, but I will not take it down, because I need it to protect myself. I will make it lower, so we can talk over it. The main issue she showed me clearly is that the wall is not the problem. The way the wall is built is the problem. As Natasja sees it, I built it alone, but I think we built a wall from both sides.

Have you built such a wall?

EMMA BENNION, UNITED KINGDOM My wall is my office at home. It is built out of nearly the same blocks as Kees's, except block 6. For me, block 6 doesn't exist, as I have done more interesting "work" since PD than before.

For many years I had no help in coming to terms with the disease, until I heard about YAPP&Rs, a young-onset support group in the UK. It was YAPP&Rs who removed block 8. So my wall is lower than Kees's, and I can climb over it when I want to. However, I don't want it taken down, as I feel safe and secure behind it, with people who really understand.

The Political Consequences of Invisibility

One of the most crucial consequences of invisibility is its negative effect on medical research funding. Politicians and government officials who allocate research funds hear patient groups who are the most vocal, the most assertive, and the most politically active. PWPs, often hampered by ravaged voices, sapped strength, and difficulty moving, were unlikely to march on Washington for a greater share of the research-funding pie. The Parkinson's community lacked a cohesive political organization and a united, loud voice in Washington, until Joan Samuelson, a young lawyer with Parkinson's, began to argue our case on Capitol Hill.

The National Institutes of Health (NIH) allocates most of the federal funding for medical research. For a decade, from 1984 to 1994, funding for PD remained stagnant, at less than $30 million dollars per year. The Parkinson's Action Network compared 1994 NIH research funding for PD with a number of other serious conditions and reported the following per patient funding amounts:

Parkinson's disease $30

Alzheimer's disease $54

Heart disease $93

Multiple sclerosis $158

Cancer $295

AIDS/HIV $1,069

By 1996, NIH direct funding for PD research increased to only $32 million, or about $32 per Parkinson's patient, continuing to be substantially lower than the amounts allocated to research for many other deadly or disabling conditions.[5]

When Joan Samuelson began knocking on doors on Capitol Hill in the early 1990s, lobbying for increased PD research funding, she noticed, "When I walked in the door it was the first time that a congressman had ever had someone visit him and talk about Parkinson's. And they'd say: 'Yeah, Parkinson's, um, yeah, that's nerves, right?' There was no awareness of what the implications of it were. There was a common belief that it's a fairly benign disorder; that we pop a pill and the symptoms go away; that it's OK."

Joan also observed, "Parkinson's patients have to blame ourselves in part for our lack of visibility. With our bravery, what we've done is render ourselves a bit invisible.... We want so badly to be out in the world, living and functioning just like everyone else. So we don't complain very much, and as a result, the American public hasn't known how awful Parkinson's is. And Congress hasn't known how awful Parkinson's is."[6]

In the years following, the Parkinson's Action Network organized a growing grassroots movement of PD advocates who pledged to be "Invisible No More." (See Chapter 6 for more about PAN.)

BARBARA PATTERSON, ONTARIO, CANADA Until and unless the devastation of Parkinson's is recognized, research into the causes/treatments/cure will continue to be underfunded. People like Janet Reno, Michael J. Fox, and Muhammad Ali are doing their share, so let's do ours. Walk for Parkinson's; talk about it; if you are fumbling for change at a checkout, explain that you have Parkinson's. I know it's easier to stay home so people won't

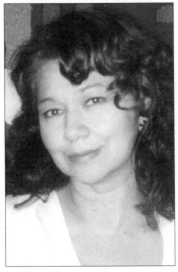

MaryHelen Davila

stare at us shaking or moving rigidly and slowly or spilling our tea, but letting them see us may inspire them to contribute to research the next time they are asked.

Tell Them

MARYHELEN DAVILA

Tell them
We're real,
We count,
We have a right to the
pursuit of happiness.
We have the right to "life"
We're not invisible...

have them look in our eyes.
We are here
We matter
We are no less than others
We won't disappear.
Tell them. Tell them again.
And Tell them again.

Lessons in Courage: Roads to Visibility

If we want the world to know our problems, we are going to have to find the courage to let the world see those problems. DENNIS GREENE

On 28 November 1998, the news wires first revealed the shocking news. A week later the cover of *People* magazine shouted from newsstands, "EXCLUSIVE—MICHAEL J. FOX—THE FIGHT OF HIS LIFE." The world learned that the popular television and movie star had been living behind a self-chosen mask for the preceding 7 years as he kept his struggles with PD hidden from the public.

Fox stated:

I had hidden my symptoms and struggles very well, through increasing amounts of medication, through surgery, and by employing the hundreds of little tricks and techniques a person with Parkinson's learns to mask his or her condition for as long as possible. While the changes in my life were profound and progressive, I kept them to myself for a number of reasons: fear, denial for sure, but I also felt that it was important for me to just quietly "soldier on."

When I did share my story, the response was overwhelming, humbling, and deeply inspiring. I heard from thousands of Americans affected by Parkinson's, writing and calling to offer encouragement and to tell me of their experience. They spoke of pain, frustration, fear, and hope. Always hope. What I understood very clearly is that the time for quietly "soldiering on" is through.[7]

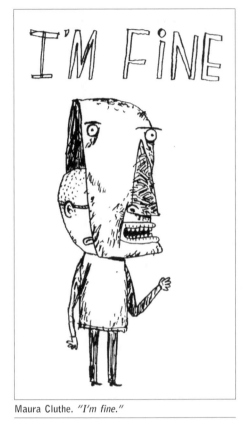

Maura Cluthe. *"I'm fine."*

Fox's courage in facing the public unmasked inspired many others to peer out from behind their masks as well. Momentarily, the existence of young people with Parkinson's drew the attention of the U.S. and world media.

Shortly after Fox's announcement, Susan Reese, coordinator of the American Parkinson Disease Association Young Onset Parkinson's Information and Referral Center, was interviewed on the *Today Show* about PD in general and about the unique problems of young-onset PWPs. A week later, Reese wrote to PIEN that the center was still "digging out from the huge number of calls that came in—and are still continuing to come in" with questions about Parkinson's disease.

ERNIE PETERS, UNITED KINGDOM I went through a period of trying to hide symptoms and avoiding telling anyone of my problem. We probably all do. Since then, I have come to the conclusion that by trying to stay invisible I was hindering the progress toward public awareness, more funding, and a possible early cure. I realize that there may be reasons why an open approach with one's employer may not be advisable, but other than that or similar circumstances, I would urge all people with PD to take opportunities to inform the public.

I am not suggesting we stand shaking on street corners with a notice around our necks. However, trying to hide our symptoms may not be in our best interest. If we struggle at the checkout or at the bank, a quick "Sorry, I have Parkinson's and it affects my movement and coordination" will not hurt. Under the right circumstances, a further few words such as "Still, I can't complain; some people with PD are confined to bed and wheelchair" are easy. Said with a smile and perhaps a joke about the handwriting, there are many instances where one more member of the public can be made aware in only a minute or so that:

- ▸ PD is nasty and progressive;
- ▸ It does not affect only old people;
- ▸ The people like me whom they meet are only the tip of the iceberg.

After all, why have a Parkinson's awareness week once a year and then go back to hiding for another 51 weeks?

LYNDA MCKENZIE I feel that it is really important to get the word about Parkinson's out to the general public. Unfortunately, as you know, most people become more reclusive when they get PD. When I did an interview on the TV program *20/20*, I was bothered at first that I was so dyskinetic, but on reflection, I realize that it was good. It showed everyone that although the results I have received from the surgery are good, it still isn't a cure. Besides, the public has to know what it's all about.

ANNE RUTHERFORD, NEWFOUNDLAND, CANADA Many years ago, I was a YOP, young-onset Parkinson. Now I am an old and tired PWP who is still trying to find the balance point between the "happy face" and a face that would terrify the most courageous person in the world. I am beginning to think the "happy face" just makes us more invisible and easier to dismiss. Tell it like it is. That's my new war cry.

RITA WEEKS, NEBRASKA We are hoping to educate the public as well as draw attention to the funding need.

We are hoping to inform patients and families who are not on the Internet or in active/well-moderated support groups.

We are hoping to educate employers to be able to understand our workplace limitations.

We need to show the truth about Parkinson's. The more we are seen at our worst, the greater the outcry for money, research, education, and aid to families.

We are hoping to educate the caregivers who are allied medical professionals and our general practitioners who are not movement-disorder specialists.

If our stories are hushed and not told, we are doing nothing to help the newly diagnosed over the current hurdle or the next hurdle.

Parkinson's is not just medication, research, and icing-on-the-cake stories. It is real life. Day-to-day coping with the change. Learning to live as a family with the change. Learning to communicate without body language. Learning to plan. Learning to accept and learning to hope. There is a heck of a lot of "stuff" the world NEEDS to know about.

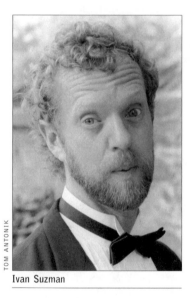

TOM ANTONIK

Ivan Suzman

IVAN SUZMAN Our faces—that is what is not being seen by the public. Morris Udall's face, lying in a hospital bed, has a vastly different impact from my face—with its relative youth, short dark beard, and pierced ear. The faces of as many of us as possible need to be seen.

Has anyone ever seen pictures sewn into panels of the AIDS quilt? The human face is so powerful, even after the soul that moved it has passed from this Earth. Please don't hide your faces. Rather a disfigured, pained, drooling face, or a masked face, than none at all. Let's see our heroes like Lonnie and Muhammad Ali, and let's also see the faces of the rest of us.

Thank you Muhammed Ali

MARYHELEN DAVILA, ARIZONA I was called yesterday by the executive director of the National Parkinson's Foundation. He said the message I e-mailed to Muhammad Ali was received, and Ali actually got it!! I only dreamed Ali might read it. I hope it makes him smile. Here it is:

July 23, 1996—Dear Muhammad Ali: I hope somehow this reaches you. Yet still, you are the greatest! You have rekindled hope for so many around the world. My daughter called me excitedly yelling, "Mom! Put the TV on. Put it on!" And as I did, I saw. . .

"In an emotional halftime ceremony [at the men's basketball finals], Muhammad Ali was given a gold medal to replace the one he no longer has from his 1960 Olympic victory. IOC president Juan Antonio Samaranch made the presentation at midcourt as the 34,600 fans roared their approval."[8]

. . . I saw you walk up and light the Olympic torch! I caught my breath as tears of admiration and gratitude for you rolled down my cheeks. I heard my daughter on the phone trying to choke back a sob. The impact of your appearance and of your lighting that marvelous torch was tremendous for us and for so many around the world who are affected by Parkinson's.

"Ali, who began these games by lighting the ceremonial torch, shuffled out to midcourt and accepted the medal from Samaranch, who kissed the boxing legend on both cheeks. Then, with one hand twitching from the ravages of Parkinson's syndrome, Ali raised the gold medal slowly to his lips and kissed it."[9]

Those who struggle to take steps, and those who no longer can, felt every step you took. We felt the same shaking and the same grip that prevents us from spontaneously cheering, waving our arms, carelessly and freely jumping and swaying and clapping like the rest of the audience watching. But your presence is a strong reminder to the world that we still feel, we still dream, and, yes, especially now—we celebrate with you the opening of the Olympic Games.

Although we cannot move, we happily celebrate with joy the magnificent and beautiful miracles of healthy competitors. The embers of our own spirit, almost smothered by Parkinsonism, sparked and burst into a beautiful flame of hope for the world to see.

"Muhammad Ali's decision to become official spokesman of the National Parkinson Foundation in the U.S., and to carry the Olympic torch at the 1996 Summer Games, drew immediate and intense attention to the disease."[10]

We want the world to see Parkinson's—we will no longer be "invisible to the world." The flame you lit represents the Olympics, but it also represents the spirit we are putting forth to fight Parkinson's. Over the years you were followed by many who were struggling but were "invisible" to the world's caregivers. Your example gives us the hope and the incentive to tough it out. To be seen. To be heard. To fight back.

"Boxing great Muhammad Ali was honored Tuesday for his fighting outside the boxing ring in his battle to vanquish Parkinson's syndrome. Ali, whose bout with the disease has left his speech slurred, used his world-renowned fame to bring the spotlight to the first national study for Parkinson's disease exclusively for minorities."[11]

And you continue.... You've done a lot for us who have Parkinson's. We've been invisible for so long, but it's time to be seen. With your help, we are not invisible anymore. With your help, Muhammad Ali, we'll knock out PD! Thank you, Muhammad Ali!

The Wish

DAVID BOOTS

The noonday sun beat down on the young man on the park bench as he twisted his body and rocked back and forth as if possessed by demons seeking to escape. His facial expressions were grimaces, and his head moved constantly like one of those dolls with the bobbing heads. His name was Chris, and at that moment, he was barely hanging on to life, wondering why all of this was happening to him.

He sat alone performing his twisted ballet, avoiding eye contact as the joggers and dog-walkers paraded past. He wasn't a junkie or a mental patient; his struggle was Parkinson's disease, and this struggle had been going on for a long time. The medicine he took was no longer effective and had turned against him, making it seem as if his limbs were being guided by a drunken puppeteer with a cruel streak.

A group of four joggers approached him as he heard one say to the others, "I'm gonna stop here and make a phone call. I'll catch up in a minute." The others responded, "See ya in a little bit, Stephen," as he stopped a few yards from Chris and got out his cell phone from his fanny pack. Chris could see that this man was in excellent shape, and he tried in vain to remember a time in his life when he had been in a similar condition. As the man sat down on the opposite end of the bench, he avoided any eye contact with Chris.

"Hi, honey, I didn't want to wake you up when I left for my run this morning. I'm going in to the office for an hour or so and then I'll meet you and the kids up at the cabin.... Yeah, take the 4x4 and bring some champagne and we'll celebrate my new promotion," he continued. Chris tried to focus on what it was like to have a job or a family or a sports-utility vehicle or a cabin to go to. His days were a nightmare of medicines, their side effects, and trying to stay near a bathroom at all times...his nights much the same.

Stephen glanced at his Rolex and felt his pulse while cradling the cell phone under his chin and looked off in the distance to avoid meeting Chris' eyes. Chris, meanwhile, was trying to reach in his pocket for his medicines and having a difficult time as uncontrollable muscle spasms rocked his upper body. He managed to get his pills out but spilled quite a few around the bench in the process. "Alright, honey. I love you, too," Stephen said as he put the phone back and stood up, crushing several of Chris' pills in the process. "Hey," Chris shouted at him, knowing how expensive his medicines were, "you're stepping on my pills."

Stephen turned to face Chris for the first time and said, "If pill-poppers like you would get off drugs and stay out of the public parks, then people like me could be free to enjoy them as they were intended. I'm tired of my tax dollars going to helping you support your habit and having you sit out here in broad daylight going through your withdrawals in front of God and everyone else." Chris replied, "I have PD...," but Stephen cut him off, saying, "PD, VD, I don't care what you call your filthy obsession, just go crawl in a hole somewhere so the world doesn't have to look at you." Chris was in shock and started to say, "I wish...," but Stephen once again cut him off and walked away muttering, "I wish decent citizens like me didn't..." as he resumed his jog.

Chris' body twisted painfully as the tears ran down his face and he said, "I wish you knew what I have to live with each day, I wish you could take this disease and deal with it for 24 hours." He lay down on the bench and began sobbing.

At that moment, Stephen's jog was cut short as his body began to twist at random in short bursts of energy. His partners were up ahead a little ways on the path but he felt something like shame wash over him and didn't try to call out. He stopped and felt something horrifying beginning. His body felt like it was trying to turn itself inside out. He had mobility and dexterity, but it was as if he had too much of each of them. His mind seemed to be racing like his body but only seemed to stop and focus on negative things, things he hadn't thought of in years. What the hell was happening?

As Chris felt his sadness quickly diminish, he was totally unprepared for what washed over him. He felt his body relax and felt the cobwebs clear from his head. He sat up straight and stretched his arms out in front of him like a cat awakening from a nap. They were both steady as a rock, something he hadn't seen in years. Something was happening to his face; he realized he was smiling. He stood up, took a deep breath, and began to run along the path, enjoying the feel of the wind on his face and the sun beating down on his skin. He knew then his wish had come true.

Stephen stopped and tried to open his fanny pack but couldn't hold still long enough to work the zipper. After much fidgeting, he finally got it open and got out his cell phone, but every time he tried to punch in a number he hit multiple keys and finally gave up in disgust. His family would soon be waiting for him at the cabin, but that seemed inconsequential compared to whatever was happening to him now. He planned on stopping at a coffee shop on the perimeter of the park to try and figure this out.

Chris was out of breath but he had so much adrenaline running through his system...he felt so alive! A Frisbee landed at his feet, and a kid's voice rang out, "Would you throw it back, mister?" Chris answered in a booming voice he hardly recognized as his own, "Go long!" as he gave it a mighty throw across the field and the child ran after it. "You certainly look like you're having a good day," said a young woman sitting on a bench nearby. Chris realized he was still grinning ear-to-ear. He had noticed her earlier on his way to the park but was too intimidated then to speak. He laughingly told her, "I really can't recall when I've felt this good," and continued on towards his apartment.

Jogging had never been this tiring and uncomfortable, Stephen thought to himself. His back hurt, his legs felt weak, and he couldn't maintain any kind of normal gait. He entered the coffee shop and sat at a table and immediately started fidgeting in his seat trying to find a posture that felt comfortable; his body seemed to have a mind of its own, as others in the shop watched him move about in his chair. He ordered a latte when the waitress came around and tried to appear normal. His jogging friends would wonder where he was, but he didn't care. He just hoped no one would recognize him. His coffee came and he spilled it on himself during his first attempted sip. Polite whispers at nearby tables told him his performance had not gone unnoticed. He ignored the stain on his jogging pants and sat there for the next hour while his mind and body spun crazily in a demented dance.

The first thing Chris did when he arrived at his place was to pick up the phone and dial a number. He hadn't made contact in years. When the voice at the other end answered, he began, "Hi, Mom, it's Chris," and then he started crying. "Oh, Chris," his mother said, " I haven't heard from you in so long. Your voice sounds so strong. Are you doing okay?" Chris said, "Mom, right now I'm having a great day. I wanted to tell you that I love you so much and that you did a wonderful job of raising all of us and that..." "Chris," his Mom interrupted, "slow down and tell me about what's happened to you." "Mom, I don't have much time. Just remember that though PD wears my body down, I'm still aware of the world around me but will simply be unable to participate any longer. I love you...always remember that," as he hung up the phone and the tears ran down his face.

The fidgeting seemed to have gone away during the hour Stephen sat trying to drink his latte without applying much more of it to his jogging outfit. Other customers came and went, so his embarrassment was kept secret from the public…until he stood up. But with the disappearance of his excess energy came a great emotional and physical drain that was pulling him down. The waitress had left him alone after cleaning two of his spills from the table and had apparently told her replacement about his odd behavior. What in the world was happening to him? One minute it felt like he had Mexican jumping beans running through his veins and now he felt like a bicycle tire slowly going flat with no visible puncture.

That afternoon, three of his old friends thought they saw a ghost as Chris ran past them in the early afternoon sun. He didn't stop to talk with any of them to try and tell them what was happening. He ordered spaghetti for lunch and handled his utensils just like old times. He couldn't stop smiling at his new gift. His gait was normal, he could smell a hundred different smells, and his lunch had tasted delicious. His senses were alive for the first time in the last 10 years.

Stephen had a difficult time getting up from the table and stumbled and lurched his way to the bathroom. His bladder didn't wait for him to make it to a stall, and the stain joined the previous coffee stains as he fought to hold his anger in check. Losing his balance, he caught himself on the wall as he clumsily fell down on the toilet seat. "What in the hell is happening to me?" he spoke aloud in the empty bathroom as tears began to run down his face. He needed to get back to his house and call a doctor and find out the cause of all this. As he left the bathroom and stumbled towards his table, one of the owners came up and said, "Listen, buddy, you need to pay up and leave." Stephen, intensely aware of his appearance, and thoroughly ashamed of his physical condition, simply nodded. His voice felt tired and he was having trouble enunciating words. At the cash register, he realized his dexterity was all but gone as he struggled to fit his hand into the wet pocket of his pants to get his wallet. After watching him struggle for several minutes, the owner said, "Just leave and don't come back," as Stephen left the coffee-house and stumbled into the late afternoon. He started back through the park towards his house.

Chris's afternoon and early-evening hours were spent downtown enjoying the hustle and bustle of city life and taking in all the sights, sounds, and smells. He went shopping for clothes and the necessary ingredients to prepare one of his favorite dishes (he couldn't remember when he had last cooked a meal on his own). He thought he saw the woman from the park at the grocery store, but he couldn't be sure and was distracted by all the wonderful smells he hadn't been aware of for years. As he made his way home, he shared his smiles with everyone he saw and was even seen skipping the final few blocks to his apartment.

The sun was setting as Stephen realized his walking (which appeared as an off-balance shuffle) wasn't going to get him home before dark. A group of youths ahead on the path looked like trouble, but Stephen's present condition allowed for neither fight nor flight, and so he continued forward, aware that his weak voice couldn't scream "Help" if he tried. His heart started racing and his hands and legs began to tremor. "That's a nice cell phone and wristwatch you got there," one of the youths said to him. Stephen mumbled, "Take anything, just please..." before the wind was knocked out of him by a fist to his stomach. He felt his bladder let go as the gang of youths removed his valuables and dragged him off the trail into the bushes, where they left him with a parting kick to his head. Everything went black.

After a wonderful dinner, Chris got out some old LPs he hadn't listened to in years and played them as he cleaned up his apartment. He had the energy of a man possessed as he brandished bucket and mop for the next several hours until it looked as clean as the day he'd moved in 10 years ago. Afterwards, he opened his window and looked out at the night sky with amazement and wondered why he hadn't done this before. He read the newspaper, filled in most of the crossword puzzle, and had a cup of tea before heading off to bed. He was asleep almost as soon as his head hit the pillow.

The automatic sprinklers woke Stephen around dawn. Through the aches and pains of the events of the night before, hunger and the need for a cup of coffee dominated his thoughts as he slowly tried to get up off the ground. His mind felt very muddled and foggy as he tried to piece together all the bizarre activity of the day before. Once standing, balance seemed a constant challenge as he stumbled down the path through the park again towards the coffee shop. Wait, he'd been kicked out yesterday afternoon, and an awkward search of his wet and dirty clothes told him that his money was gone too. The bench ahead of him looked familiar as he lurched towards it and plopped down. As he sat with his hands and legs shaking uncontrollably and a depressing movie playing continuously on a big screen inside his head, he tried to remember what had instigated all of this...an altercation of some sort. Then he saw the pills on the ground at his feet, and as he picked the pieces off the ground a dim lightbulb went on in his head.

Chris couldn't remember a better night's sleep in his life. He thought of making an omelet but decided to dress up in his new clothes and go out for brunch. He went to a small restaurant downtown that he had heard served wonderful breakfasts (his PD had never allowed him to eat comfortably in front of others). His meal was better than he imagined, and he was having champagne and orange juice as an after-meal treat when he spotted her: the woman from the park yesterday that he thought he'd seen at the grocery store. She was heading toward the same spot in the park as before, so Chris finished his drink, paid his bill, and headed into the park looking for her.

Stephen sat looking at the pieces of yellow and brown pills in his hand as he replayed the events of yesterday in his mind. The pill-popping fellow on the bench yesterday had become upset when some of his pills had been stepped on. Hadn't he had something physical going on that looked like what Stephen was enduring? His brain was muddled and he wasn't sure anymore. He clutched the pieces tightly in his hand as the morning park crowd began to parade past his bench, trying not to stare at his horrible appearance and his trembling extremities. Thinking he had nothing to lose, Stephen swallowed the hodge-podge of pills and waited for something to happen.

Chris saw her near the grassy field, sitting and people-watching. "Hello," she said when she saw him. "Having another good day?" Chris smiled as he sat down. He asked her, "Would you like to hear a story?" "Sure," she replied.

Chris proceeded to tell her of a man who was banished from participating in everyday life and who was forced to carry his prison cell with him everywhere he went. But one day, as he was watching the people laugh and point at him, he made a wish. Chris paused as she asked, "What was the wish?" He told her that the man wished to be set free just for the day while one of his tormentors took his place. He paused again as she asked, "So what happened to both of them?" Chris glanced at his watch and said "Look, it's been a pleasure talking to you like this. I've got to run right now. Next time I see you, I'll fill you in on the rest of the story." With a vague idea of what was to happen next, Chris headed for the bench where it had all started yesterday. He was not prepared for what awaited him there.

As he sat the on the bench for the next 45 minutes, Stephen felt his mind clear as his limbs started to cooperate with him. "This has been sort of bad dream," he said aloud to no one as life once again began to flow through his system. But the longer he sat there, the more nervous excess energy began to take over. Like yesterday's experience, but worse, he thought as he began to squirm and twist on the bench. "Oh God, here we go again," he cried as the movements became more exaggerated. And then he spotted Chris.

Still excited from talking to the woman he'd been so intimidated by in the past, Chris was almost to the bench before he spotted Stephen squirming and fidgeting in his stained jogging outfit from yesterday. "Did you have a nice day?" Chris taunted as he sat down next to him. Then, noticing some yellow and brown pieces around Stephen's mouth, Chris asked sternly, "How much did you take and how long ago?" Stephen replied that he'd taken the pills that had fallen to the ground yesterday when they encountered one another. Chris asked, "All of them?" to which Stephen nodded yes as his movements increased. "Now, you know how bad PD is, don't you? Are you going to be rude again to someone you see shuffling or trembling?" Chris barked at him. Stephen just said, "I'm so sorry...I didn't know," as tears filled his eyes and his body attempted to turn itself inside out.

Chris had been away from his medicine for 24 hours and a feeling of doom and gloom clamped down over his mind as he watched Stephen's body suddenly relax and his facial features soften. Stephen, his body awakened from his bad dream, got up quickly off the bench and started running towards his house with no further words to Chris. He'd call his family, since they were certainly wondering where he'd gone to, and get cleaned up out of this mess he was wearing. He couldn't believe what he had just gone through and prayed it would never happen again. Some friends called out to him as he ran past, but one look at his appearance was enough to frighten children and small animals and he continued on.

Chris was so weak that he couldn't get up right away. His medicine was back at the apartment, but that seemed a lifetime away in terms of available energy. He began to shuffle and stumble down the path towards his apartment when he spotted her. It was too late to go another way and so without looking in her direction, he kept going.

She was shocked to see the fellow who had left her not too long ago in the middle of telling her a story stumbling down the path towards her. He acted as if he didn't want her to notice him, but the tears rolling down his cheeks and his awkward gait told her what a difficult time he was having.

"Hey," she said, her voice catching, "I'd like to hear the rest of your story sometime." Chris said, "Are you sure?" She looked at him for a second and stood up and walked over to him. As she took his hand, she said, "Sure, I've got all the time in the world," as they walked along. She had decided that good people like this are rare and that she wanted to be part of a story that never ends.[12]

chapter 6

"Invisible No More!": Empowerment Through Community

ALAN BONANDER DIED in early August 1996. Many on the Parkinson's Information Exchange Network (PIEN) expressed their personal loss, although most had never actually met him in person. Alan was known to us by his advice and friendship offered through e-mail and his postings to the list. A 12-year veteran of living with and fighting PD, including a pallidotomy in Sweden, the 56-year-old activist succumbed to asthma.[1]

DON BERNS, PENNSYLVANIA   Your computer control room lined with books, handouts, computer screens, and diskettes made an indelible impression on me. From within this room poured forth so much wisdom and compassion, along with a wry sense of humor. I remember the gracious hospitality I received when I stayed in the Bonander home from you and your delightful wife, Jane.

I remember those two days in your home being amazed at all the people who sought out your counsel by telephone. You were absolutely gracious and compassionate in dealing with a newly diagnosed Parkinson's patient who would call late at night, all the while an informed patient advocate when it came to dealing with the medical community, unafraid to take on doctors who were uninformed or misinformed concerning the treatment of Parkinson's disease. Always interested in the latest research developments, you kept many of us up to speed.

In your last year as president of the Young Onset Parkinson's Group, you hosted the statewide Parkinson's Movers and Shakers meeting in San Mateo. I will always remember you as a person of incredible energy, with glasses slipping down your nose, vest unbuttoned, perspiration beading on your brow as you emceed the meeting with diplomacy and grace.

Thanks, Alan, for sharing your life so openly and courageously with us. Your community spirit serves as an inspiration to all of us—doctors, neurologists, neurosurgeons, researchers, senators, representatives, patients, and caregivers—to ease the burden and find a cure.

Unleashing the Human Spirit via the Internet

The Parkinson's Information and Exchange Network (PIEN) was created by Barbara Patterson of Hamilton, Canada, on 8 November 1993. Within 5 days, there were 46 subscribers from Austria, France, Brazil, South Africa, Canada, and the United States. Within a year, there were 308 members from 18 countries, and as of March 2001, reflecting the unbounded growth of the Internet as a means of communication and information, there were 2,000 subscribers from 37 nations.

BARBARA PATTERSON, ONTARIO, CANADA ("LIST MOM")
Never, in the known history of this planet, has this kind of relationship existed. We meet in a place that has no walls. We talk to our friends whom we have never seen. We care deeply for other members whom we will never physically hug....

I have always felt that we hear each other better on the list because we can't see each other. Symptoms, age, color, race don't interfere. The list knows no countries, has nothing to do with money; there's no "what's in it for me."

TIM HODGENS, PSYCHOLOGIST, MASSACHUSETTS When I first saw people with Parkinson's disease, I saw the mask. When I joined the Parkinson's list, I saw people beyond the mask. The keyboard and the Internet have brought people together. This is cutting down on the isolation, but it is also showing all that is within, that ordinarily is not shown outside.

JERRY FINCH, TEXAS The impact of the Internet will be felt by all of us. We are going to find that this is truly a global village. Our interaction with one another, our methods of doing business, our realm of knowledge is now changing and will continue to change.

Ten years ago, many PWPs were no doubt very isolated. Today, just by placing one's page on the net, one can reach out to family and friends, and they, in turn, can reach him. Our common PD might still keep us from physically wandering too far, but through our computer we can reach the far ends of the earth. We are no longer alone; that's a wonderful feeling.

JUDITH RICHARDS, ONTARIO, CANADA After several visits to a psychiatrist and mounds of Kleenex, I began to realize that my life wasn't over. I discovered the Internet. I joined the PIEN, met and made friends with Parkinsonians and their care partners all over the world. As I talked to them and learned, I discovered I was still able to help others. I still had something to offer.

The first real contact I made was with a man in Rhode Island. He was going to have a pallidotomy and had run into problems with a medication he was taking. I wrote to him about drug sensitivity, and we have been friends ever since.

The Internet has provided me with the opportunity to feel useful again. As well as joining the Parkinson list, I began searching the Net for information about Parkinson's, and I was amazed by the amount of information I was able to easily access from my home. The information I found was too good to keep to myself, and I began sending these articles to the Parkinson list.

MARGARET TUCHMAN, NEW JERSEY How do I fit into this living organism? I continue to grow as a person, draw strength from the collective energy, and try to give back information and most definitely affection to the members. Discovering the Internet as a tool and the people as an extended family keeps me interested and active.

SONIA NIELSEN, DENMARK   Dear listfriends :-)) (means a big smile)

Here in Denmark, it is the early morning. I start my day taking my first dose of medicine. Next step is to open my computer and look for new e-mail. Even if I'm stiff, I use my fingers to type, use my brain to think, try to use my English, and most important, I have some wonderful people to share my thoughts and feelings with. I can laugh with you, cry with you, share my feelings with you. If I haven't seen a member for some weeks, I'm worried, but suddenly that person is "onboard" again. In my opinion every subject is important, because it is important to the person who wrote to the list. I have often done so in the middle of the night when I couldn't sleep.

"Tell Me More!": 24 Hours on the Parkinson's List

The following is typical of a newbie's (new member's) first encounter on the Parkinson's list—many questions, many fears for the future. Welcomes, answers, and cyber-hugs are shared, sometimes within minutes. There is also a spiraling effect—as newbies gain knowledge and experience living with PD, some take on the roles of welcomers and information providers. Many long-lasting friendships have resulted from that first "Tell me more!"

September 17, 3:39 P.M.
From: Sherry Macredes
Subject: Tell me more!

I am a 47-year-old female who has just been diagnosed with PD. So far, I cannot use my left hand very well and get shakes when I try. My left leg is also starting to get the jittery feeling. Also, there is the problem with rigid muscles, which is the worst!

I guess I don't have much to complain about except lack of information. The doctors (and I have seen many) don't seem to want to give you any info. I am starting the drug pramipexole and am having some difficulty with nausea, but since the dose is still not enough, I haven't gotten any relief from my symptoms.

Do any of you know anything about this drug and what I can expect? I have read everything I can find on the Web, but it is just too depressing. The doctors say, don't worry, you should have many years of productive living.

What can I really expect? How long will I be able to continue to work? I do accounting and use the keyboard a lot, which is getting very hard to do. Should I be planning for assisted care soon? I know these questions are unanswerable, but I wish someone could give me a ballpark figure...say, "5 to 10 years before you will require help with daily chores"—or something!

I'm sure all of you went through this period of confusion.

During the day, my husband and I discuss where we will put our backpacks on the next road trip; at night alone in my thoughts I wonder where we will put my wheelchair. I would appreciate any answers to unanswerable questions. Thanks.

4:55 P.M.
From: Charles Meyer

Sherry,

I am a 54-year-old physician (psychiatrist), retired because of PD about 2½ years ago. I was diagnosed at age 44 and continued practicing until I was about 52. But things are getting better. Medications may slow the progress of the disease, and if that doesn't work as far as symptoms go, there is always the gold standard, levodopa, which will almost certainly bring you back to near normal. Also, there are surgeries that are being improved on all the time, such as deep brain stimulation, which are helpful if and when you reach that point. While PD is an awful disease, the cure is not far off, so it is my hope that you and I will see it, and hopefully before you get significantly debilitated.

Regarding doctors, I suggest that you at least consult with a movement-disorders specialist. Unfortunately, there are many M.D.s who don't know about the latest trends in PD care and may treat you as they were trained 10 or 15 years ago.

Good luck, and please feel free to e-mail me at any time.

5:17 P.M.
From: Sandra Norris

I am a 39-year-old woman who has had PD since the age of 20. I was finally properly diagnosed at the age of 28. When the diagnosis came, I was already wheelchair-bound and in the care of my parents. I was totally disabled. But the good news is when I was on the proper medicinal program and had the right neurologists, I was able to walk again and live on my own. I now use a wheelchair maybe one to two times a week. I live alone and try my best to help others with this horrible illness.

I wish I had specific answers to your questions or even answers that you "want" to hear. If I am understanding, your main battle right now is coping...understanding...living with this disease. You will need to find a neurologist that you feel comfortable with and trust. A good medicinal program is important as well. Of course, support groups and love and understanding from friends and family will help too. I will tell you this: you are not alone, although that is really how you feel right now. If there is anything I can help you with, please feel free to e-mail me.

8:40 P.M.
From: Linda Greulich

I was officially diagnosed in August 1994, and like so many, I had symptoms for some years prior to diagnosis. I was 45 at the time.

This list has played a very important part in my attitude, education, and decision making. The most important benefit of this list for me has been education! The saying that knowledge is power in this case is very appropriate. I have learned so much, and that learning has opened the door to better relationships with my doctors. I continue to educate them. I agree with Barbara Patterson when she said the most knowledgeable will live the longest!

September 18, 12:38 A.M.
From: Sharon Habing

I think it is really important to find a doctor whose specialty is movement disorders. We drive 2 hours to get to mine. For free literature, contact the National Parkinson Foundation and the American Parkinson Disease Association. Tell them you are newly diagnosed and ask them to send you any and all booklets, brochures, etc., that are available. There is also the APDA Young Parkinson's Information and Referral Center. Ask them to send you *The Young Parkinson's Handbook*, and if you have children, ask them about PDKIDS. [See the resource guide for information about these organizations.]

4:00 P.M.
From: Sherry Macredes

Thanks to you who have responded to my questions. This is the first time I have actually talked about my PD with anyone, and after the initial typing through the tears, I realize I am not alone at all. There are a lot of people who have coped well with this disease and are really living their lives. Somehow, that makes it easier for me. You have answered my questions and offered suggestions that no one else has been able to do. Thanks to all of you, and keep hanging in there. I hope someday to be able to help others in the way you have helped me.

A Global Conversation on Nutrition

Kathrynne Holden is a registered dietitian and a pioneer in the field of nutrition and Parkinson's disease. She has authored two books (see the resource guide, Appendix 2) and various journal articles, and she has lectured around the world. Kathrynne is also a longtime member of PIEN; she donates her time and expertise answering the many questions posted to the list about nutrition and diet.

Joy Graham is a caregiver for her husband, Bob, and a committee member of the Parkinson's Association of Western Australia. Joy and Bob became familiar with Kathrynne and her work on the PIEN list and played a key role in helping Kathrynne educate other nutritionists and PWPs throughout the global community.

JOY GRAHAM, AUSTRALIA It might seem mysterious as to why we in Perth should have anything to do with Kathrynne in

Colorado; however, when we invited Kathrynne to speak at the conference in Perth, she had already proved herself as someone who really knew about PD and nutrition. I had been "listening" and "observing" her responses to the list for a long time before we issued the invitation.

KATHRYNNE HOLDEN, COLORADO The PD listserv has been, and is, a big part of my life. It has helped increase my understanding of nutrition in PD and my commitment to enhancing the awareness of Parkinson's disease in other health professionals.

Although nutrition cannot provide a cure for PD, it is my belief that many PD-related hospitalizations are nutrition related and are mostly preventable. As a result, I wrote a handbook, *Eat Well, Stay Well with Parkinson's Disease.*

(See the resource guide, Appendix 2, for information about books by Kathrynne Holden.)

JOY GRAHAM When Kathrynne confirmed that she was coming, she set about getting the e-mails and addresses of local nutritionists so she could talk to them. In both Sydney and Perth, she addressed students and professionals, and in Perth she went on the radio and gave a superb talk about nutrition and PD. She did all this unfunded and gave up the better part of her holiday time.

KATHRYNNE HOLDEN I have also been asked to write a professional manual on nutrition and PD for dietetics practitioners. I have submitted my study for publication in the *Journal of the American Dietetic Association.* Two state dietetic associations have asked me to speak on nutrition and PD at the annual meetings next year. This is a breakthrough into a previously little-known area. I hope it will spark further studies and research among others.

This has all come together since I returned from speaking at the PD conference in Perth. So, it would be true to say that Joy and Bob Graham are in great part responsible for this furtherance of awareness of nutrition and PD.

Thoughts on Meeting a "Cyber-Sis" in Person

SANDRA NORRIS, NORTH CAROLINA

Dear Joan [Snyder],

There is no way that I will ever be able to describe all this week has meant to me. I feel as though I have an extended family here in Chillicothe. Your family and friends opened their hearts and their homes to me as if they had known me all of my life. I enjoyed meeting and getting to know them. I guess it is the common thread of Parkinson's disease that brought us together and the common bond of love that knits us together.

It was an awakening experience—almost like gazing into a mirror, looking upon oneself but seeing into another person's soul. To know that someone else is experiencing the same challenges, triumphs, and, of course, heartache and pain that come with living with Parkinson's disease seemed to comfort my heart. Not that I would wish for anyone to suffer from PD, but knowing there are PWPs out there striving for a common goal and willing to help one another overcome, just for one day, the madness of this disease has literally caused my heart and mind to be moved beyond words.

Support Groups

One of the most influential factors in quality of life for PWPs is access to and involvement in a support group. Yet many find it very difficult to attend that first meeting for fear of seeing others in more advanced stages of the disease—and perhaps their own future. Many younger PWPs do not have local support groups specifically for people their own age and may feel uncomfortable in a group of much older members. However, searching for a support group you feel comfortable with, or starting your own, is well worth the effort. Many PD organizations will help locate groups, and there are support-group databases available on the Web. (See the resource guide.)

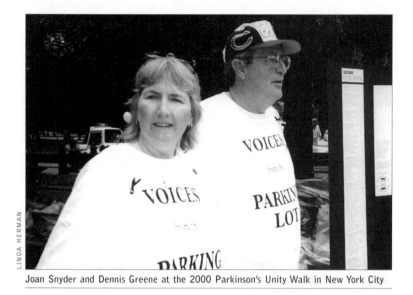

LINDA HERMAN

Joan Snyder and Dennis Greene at the 2000 Parkinson's Unity Walk in New York City

BLAIR ASHWORTH, UNITED KINGDOM I'm...reluctant to meet other sufferers, because I don't want the only thing we have in common to be a condition.... Meeting someone who's in a more advanced stage frightens me, because I know it will be like looking into the future, and I'm not quite ready for that.[2]

CELIA JONES, AUSTRALIA I feel ambiguous about being a member of Parkinson's support groups because I see my future problems reflected in those who are in more advanced stages than I. It frightens me that my symptoms are now becoming more visible, that people might now be thinking when they see me what I used to think about other PWPs.

However, when I'm in a room with other PWPs, there is also a closeness and acceptance of each other, as we can relate to each other's problems, share solutions, and offer friendship on a much deeper level than the usual acquaintances we make in daily life. The goals of a good support group should not, however, just focus on the effects of Parkinson's, but should also give purpose and encouragement to its members to look beyond the physical manifestations to the real self underneath. We are not just our disease.

DAVID BOOTS, CALIFORNIA The first PD support group I attended was disappointing and depressing. I walked in with a hope that this group of people and I could connect, and I greeted them with "What's shaking?" No one even smiled (masks?). Their presentation that day was about living wills and using walkers. I wanted to talk about PD and its effect on dating and roller skating.

MARGE SWINDLER, KANSAS We found a young-onset support group to be a lifesaver. The issues are indeed very different when you're dealing with employment, young families, sex, sports and physical activities, and planning for the future—when you're looking at supporting yourself or your family for many, many years, yet you know that your working years will be cut short.

EMMA BENNION, UNITED KINGDOM The original young-onset support group was YAPP&Rs (Young Alert Parkinson's Partners and Relatives) in the United Kingdom. The idea was put to Mary Baker, who was then the welfare director of the Parkinson's Disease Society of the UK, and as the result of several weekend seminars, the special-interest group YAPP&Rs was born. Since then, many groups for young-onset PWPs have formed around the world.[3]

...New Zealand, Australia, Denmark, Holland, France, Germany, Sweden, Kenya, Belgium, the United States, and many more. We were the first to host the Euro YAPmeet and would love to host what I believe could be the first World YAPmeet.

DIETMAR WESSEL, GERMANY I am member of the German PD association (DPV—15,000 members). Under its roof, the few younger PD patients have formed the "Club U 40" (outbreak of PD under 40). We are organized in a few regional groups and hold seminars and social gatherings. My own participation is limited so far to a weekend seminar where I met other younger patients. My family (we have two kids) joined the seminar and were, for the first time, confronted with the various stages of PD. It was interesting and encouraging to share views on PD and to learn about PD research.

ALAN RICHARDS, ONTARIO, CANADA There's a Parkinson's partners' support group here in London, Ontario, which meets in the afternoon once a month. Besides giving us an opportunity to compare notes with other caregivers, it gives us a break from the chores of caring for our partners with PD. But best of all, it's where I learned some of the things I know now. For instance:

- It's not unusual for a Parkinsonian's moods to change without notice.
- It's not a good idea to pepper them with questions when they're "off."
- Satin sheets make it easier for a Parkinsonian to turn over in bed, but don't wear silk pajamas at the same time or you might slide right out of bed. (It happened!)

It's very rewarding to be able to help your loved ones realize they *can* do more things than they *can't* do. Some of these things I was already learning by trial and error, but having other partners talk about similar situations made me realize that others had been there, done that, and they either had suggestions or sympathy for me.

JUDITH RICHARDS In the nearly 6 years that Al and I have been living with Parkinson's, we have learned that the secret of coping with Parkinson's or any chronic illness is attitude—positive attitude. Joining a support group where you can talk to others who share your concerns, joys, and sorrows is probably one of the most important things you can do to keep a positive outlook.

The Power of Community: Political Advocacy

While Mo Udall lay silent and isolated in his private room at the VA Hospital, the walls covered with photos from his pro basketball days, presidential campaign posters, and other political mementos, hopes for funding the cure energized other PWPs to become politically active, often for the first time in their lives. By speaking out and facing the world unmasked, many also found their true selves again.

The Parkinson's Action Network (PAN)

Joan Samuelson met Anne Udall, Mo's daughter, at a 1991 congressional hearing on legislation to lift the ban on federal funding of fetal-tissue transplant research. Before his fall, Mo had considered a fetal-tissue transplant, which had shown promising experimental results in combating Parkinson's disease. Anne and Joan soon became close allies against obstacles they found blocking the progress of Parkinson's research.

As they contacted Parkinson's groups throughout the country, they learned that there was little political advocacy taking place. Joan and Anne, aware of the funding successes of other, politically visible patient groups, such as AIDS activists and breast cancer survivors, came to believe that PWPs must also be "Invisible No More." Guided by this motto, Joan founded the Parkinson's Action Network (PAN) in 1991 to be a strong political voice of Parkinson-afflicted Americans, and Anne became chairman of the board.

PAN's first mission was to support the campaign for federal funding of fetal-tissue research. A bill ending the ban was passed in the House in 1991 and in the Senate in March 1992, but was vetoed by President George Bush. The House then failed by 12 votes to override the veto.

President Bill Clinton lifted the ban in 1993, as one of his first acts as president. As he signed his executive order, Clinton held up his pen and remarked, "This is for you, Mo."[4]

Four years later, Clinton signed another measure, named in honor of Morris Udall. Among the guests invited to the Oval Office to witness this signing were Joan Samuelson, Norma Udall, Mo's widow, and Jim Cordy, a retired engineer from Pittsburgh known as "The General" for his role in organizing a unique electronic grassroots campaign.

Political Activism on the Internet

TIM HODGENS One enormously powerful consequence of the Internet has been the grassroots political activism that it has fostered. This is a wonderful development, which in my humble opinion needs to be taken further. By "further" I mean a combination of political activism and of "coming out" from behind the mask of anonymity.

KEN AIDEKMAN, NEW JERSEY   My first contact with PD advocacy was through Ken Bernstein of the Young Onset Parkinson's Support Group of Massachusetts. Ken gave me information about a Parkinson's group that posted messages on a Prodigy bulletin board. Not long after that, America Online had its own "folder" for posting messages. Ken Bernstein envisioned a vast network of grassroots PWPs using the Internet to spread important stories to many groups for their newsletters.

Ken told me about Alan Bonander and the great things he was doing on the West Coast. I met Alan via Prodigy. He was immediately friendly and helpful.

As the Parkinson Information Exchange Network (PIEN) continued to grow in membership, news of the mailing list began to spread on the Internet to other computer enthusiasts. By 1994, news of legislative initiatives and public-awareness events were posted on PIEN and other Internet sites. Ken Bernstein's vision of a grassroots political network for PWPs was becoming a reality.

An Electronic Grassroots Campaign

On 24 July 1994, Alan Bonander sent the following announcement, written by Ken Aidekman, to PIEN:

I am passing on information from the AOL Parkinson's Disease Bulletin Board. On July 19th, Senator Mark O. Hatfield (R-OR) and Congressman Henry A. Waxman (D-CA) introduced the Morris K. Udall Parkinson's Research, Education and Assistance Act of 1994.

The Morris K. Udall Act will:

► Expand basic and clinical research into Parkinson's, and coordinate the research agenda;
► Establish Parkinson's research centers across the country;
► Establish Morris K. Udall Excellence Awards and feasibility study grants;

- Establish patient and family registries;
- Establish Morris K. Udall Health Professions training grants; and
- Establish a National Parkinson's Disease Education Program.

The congressmen present spoke of their personal experiences with Parkinson's.... Senator Paul Wellstone emotionally affirmed his commitment to Parkinson's research while acknowledging that both of his parents suffered from the disease. Congressman Fred Upton was visibly moved as he recalled the experience of his uncle's battle with Parkinson's.

"Parkinson's has not had a significant breakthrough in treatment since the development of L-dopa in the sixties," said Joan Samuelson, president of PAN. "Scientists tell us a major breakthrough and even the cure can be found...if their research is supported. Unfortunately, Parkinson's has been the stepchild of the federal budget. With this bill, the neglect of our community will begin to end."

A Call to Arms

The PIEN became a valuable tool for sharing information about the Udall Bill and strategies for achieving its passage. Over the following four years, list members joined others from all over the United States to lobby their representatives and senators by phone, by mail, and in person to amass support for the Udall Bill. PWPs from around the globe, inspired by the activism demonstrated by their American counterparts, began organizing similar initiatives in their own countries. The dedication and perseverance of people like Jim Cordy inspired many on the PIEN to answer his "Call to Arms."

JIM CORDY, PENNSYLVANIA Greetings, I'm sending this out to a list of names I have collected over the past year or so. Some of you I know well. Some of you I do not know at all, but have simply been intrigued by something you posted on the PIEN list, some tone in your message that I thought indicated that you might want to participate in this effort to cure Parkinson's disease.

I titled this message "Call to Arms." We need each of you and all the additional support you can muster to provide a massive grassroots demand to pass the Udall Bill. At stake is the

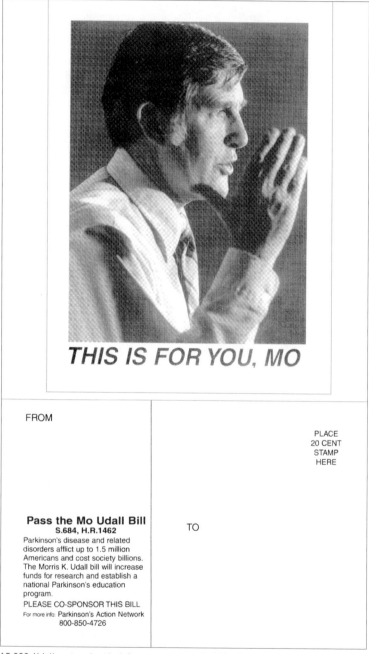

THIS IS FOR YOU, MO

FROM

PLACE
20 CENT
STAMP
HERE

Pass the Mo Udall Bill
S.684, H.R.1462

TO

Parkinson's disease and related
disorders afflict up to 1.5 million
Americans and cost society billions.
The Morris K. Udall bill will increase
funds for research and establish a
national Parkinson's education
program.
PLEASE CO-SPONSOR THIS BILL
For more info: Parkinson's Action Network
800-850-4726

DESIGNED BY KEN AIDEKMAN

65,000 Udall postcards asked Congress to pass the Udall Bill — "Do it for Mo" potential of cutting years off the time it will take to cure Parkinson's disease. That is what this call to arms is about. We must identify advocates, train them, arm them with the facts, and convince them that they can make a difference.

If we had one person with Parkinson's disease personally visit each senator and representative, we would get this Udall Bill passed.

PIEN Members Answer the Call

Among those who answered the call were Barbara Schirloff of New Jersey, who printed and distributed 65,000 postcards to be sent to Congress in support of the Udall Bill; Bob Dolezal and MaryHelen Davila of Arizona, whose perseverance won over an important ally in the Senate; and Gail Vass of Virginia, who learned that we can all make a difference.

In a letter to the authors, Barbara Schirloff related the story behind her postcard campaign to sign up congressional sponsors for the Udall Bill:

Ken Aidekman created, designed and printed up the original Udall postcards as a means of helping people contact their congressmen without having to write a letter. I was flabbergasted at the simplicity of his idea, yet with such enormous potential. I thought they should be distributed across the country to every support group or person with an interest in PD.

I started by getting 5,000 postcards printed (at the time, one of my brothers was able to get it done for free) and wrote to the PIEN list about distributing free Udall postcards to anyone who would send them to their congressional representatives. I also tried to provide the names and addresses of their representatives, along with additional members of Congress who were targeted because of their committee seats. At Jim Cordy's suggestion, I also provided preaddressed labels.

I used grocery money up front, and continued as long as I could, asking people just to send back the postage. After 50,000 postcards were printed, Margaret Tuchman (another list member) offered to help financially...and to help me send out the postcards, because orders were coming in fast and furious.

THE GOAL: One postcard from every Parkinson's patient, every caregiver, every husband, every wife, every brother or sister, every significant other, every child and grandchild, every doctor, every receptionist or nurse or pharmacist, every other person who can sign their name.

THE RESULTS: The Udall postcards went like wildfire. A total of 65,000 postcards were printed and distributed, some as far away as Hawaii and Australia. While we don't know the exact number delivered to Capitol Hill, we know the postcards were explosively effective en masse in boosting support for the Udall Bill.

The following, written by PIEN list member Bob Dolezal, originally appeared as a "Guest Comment" in the *Arizona Daily Star* in July 1996:

We were in Washington, about three dozen of us, to convince the Congress to pass and appropriate funds for the Morris K. Udall Parkinson's Research Act....

A few of the "advocates" were not Parkinsonian—Brad Udall, Mo's son, was one—but most of us were. Many, now in their 30s and 40s, had been visited by this insidious and incurable disease far earlier in life's "normal" cycle than I. Many suffered from frequent tremors, unsteady walk and minced steps, muted voice, soreness and fatigue and falling. But all were eager to take on their "mission impossible."

I was to join MaryHelen Davila from Phoenix and Brad to meet with staff in the offices of Senators John McCain and Jon Kyl, neither a co-sponsor of the bill. For eight months, my Parkinson's Advocates Committee had inundated Sen. McCain with letters and analyses, including a write-in/call-in campaign involving over a thousand people.... With NIH tacitly opposing the bill, he would not sign on as a co-sponsor....

"The senator supports Parkinson's research," an aide intoned. "But he doesn't want to tell the NIH what to do."

I noticed tears welling in MaryHelen's eyes. About then the door to Sen. McCain's private office opened, he appeared, alone, jacketless, and walked directly to our table. He wanted to meet us, he said, to express his appreciation for our long trip to see him, and just to say hello.

His entry seemed to surprise everyone, including staff. If ever *carpe diem* applied, I thought, it is now. "You are CEO of a corporation, Senator," I began, "and a team of experts tells you that by investing one hundred million dollars a year for five years you will significantly reduce overhead of fifty-six billion dollars annually. You'll take a look, won't you? Well, that's what many researchers in Parkinson's say the Udall funds can do for America."

He listened, nodded, and looked at Brad. "You sure bear a close resemblance to your dad," he said. Brad thanked him, and then, really resembling his father, suggested that Congress, rather than being reluctant to intervene, should be involved in NIH funding decisions, like a board of directors.

Next MaryHelen spoke of those unable to be present. "We're here for so many, who can't use a phone, write, can't even get up, like Brad's dad...." Exhausted, MaryHelen whispered to the senator, "I've had it seven years, I'm almost out of time. I just don't want to linger, requiring care for decades, helpless."

The senator glanced at Brad. "I have to go see Mo real soon. It's been far too long." It was said to himself more than to us. An uneasy silence settled over the group. What more was there to say?...

Then, with barely a pause, "I'll co-sponsor the bill."... Just like that. Seven months of frustration and I get to hear it from Sen. McCain himself....

I began to cry. Tears rolled down my cheeks.... MaryHelen matched me, tear for tear. Brad, looking even more like Mo, smiled broadly. The two staffers sat mute, in disbelief. I'm not sure, but I think Sen. McCain was a bit surprised, too. I rose, extended my hand, and muttered through the tears, "Thank you, Senator."...

We don't know when, or why, John McCain decided to do what he did. For eight months, his staff and I had been at a standoff. What had changed? Had he just recently become aware of us? Was it the realization of the inequities in funding? Was it Mo, a man he revered, his presence visited by a son? Or, Mary-Helen's poignant appeal?

Probably it was all those things. But most important, I believe, was that we had personally come here to make our case, advocates for a just cause.[5]

GAIL VASS, VIRGINIA My sister Edna Earle has PD. It broke my heart. I read the posts on the Udall Bill and all the political talk. I worked on a letter to ask my representative for support. I asked my family members if they wanted to read and sign one for themselves. They were VERY EAGER. I got requests for more copies for friends.

I then decided to take a bunch (already stamped) to our Young PD support group. Some had difficulty even writing their name, much less writing a letter. Everyone signed a letter and expressed appreciation for giving them an opportunity to join in the fight.

When I realized how everyone wanted to help, I sent them to my mother for her to take to her church and neighbors since they were in my representative's district.

She had so many signed letters to send that my sister Edna told her to take them to the congressman's office. She did so, and his staff paid attention to her and her concern for her daughter's future. Edna and Perry Cohen then urged Mom to ask for and get a meeting with the congressman to personally address her concerns. Mom, Edna, and Perry attended the meeting.

I've never seen our political system work; I've never wanted to be involved in the political process; I never thought a person could make a difference in the giant scheme of things; I'm stunned at the results I've seen.

AUTHORS' NOTE: *As a direct result of this family's efforts, Representative Bliley, chair of the crucial House Commerce Committee, agreed to hold hearings on the Udall Bill.*

It's Official—Udall Bill Becomes Law!

On 13 November 1997, Michael Claeys, of the Parkinson's Action Network, posted the following victory message to the PIEN:

After an intensive four-year campaign, the Udall Bill, the nation's first legislation specifically focused on Parkinson's research, has now become the law of the land. To pursue a cure, the Udall Bill *authorizes* the National Institutes of Health (NIH) to devote up to one hundred million dollars for research focused on

Parkinson's in 1998, and such sums as necessary in 1999 and 2000, [and to]:

▶ establish up to ten Udall Parkinson's Research Centers...for training, public education, and data collection;

▶ establish Udall Awards for Excellence for individual investigators with records of innovation and achievement in Parkinson's research;

▶ establish an information clearinghouse for demographic and statistical data on Parkinson's patients.

The grassroots community deserves tremendous credit for all their hard work—from writing letters to lobbying in the halls of Congress to providing the strength and momentum that led to today's celebration.

JIM CORDY

Thanksgiving 1997

Today I'm stepping out of my battle armor to bask in the glory of our great victory. I marvel at the strength of the bonds of friendship that have formed so quickly. I thought once I would never have friendships as strong as those I formed in the cauldron of my college career. But I see it is the experience of being thrown together, sharing the same vulnerability and purpose, that is the main ingredient.

From seeing those who had lost hope share in my conviction, to the signing of each and every additional cosponsor, to witnessing each deliberate stroke with fifty pens as the president of the United States of America signed into law one hundred million dollars per year for battle against Parkinson's.

I'm thankful for this list, which has enabled the connection of so many people, thoughts, and ideas. Those who have doubts about computer technology should have witnessed the Udall saga unfold post by post. There were no junkets, PACs, or high-priced lobbyists. Instead, there were letters, postcards, phone calls, and visits by ordinary people.

PD Activism Goes Global

In 1998, Ana Mari del Arco, a Spanish Parkinson patient, began contacting members of the European Parliament about the low funding of Parkinson's research in Europe. She sought to also raise awareness in the European community about the lives of the one million Europeans struggling with Parkinson's disease, similar to Joan Samuelson's campaign in the United States.

Through a French-language mailing list for Parkinson's patients, Ana Mari networked with other PWPs—Béenédicte Boutet from France, Jeremy Browne from the United Kingdom, and Dietmar Wessel from Germany—to create EUROPARK, a new advocacy organization for European Parkinsonians.

The Politics of Medical Research Funding

For the two years following the Udall Act's passage, Congress was hesitant to "earmark" or dictate funding to the National Institutes of Health for specific diseases. Therefore, the one hundred million dollars *authorized* by the Udall Act was not *appropriated* to the NIH; that is, the NIH was not given the money by Congress to spend specifically for PD research. Seasoned Parkinson's activists intensified their lobbying efforts to achieve full funding of the Udall Act, and they were joined by some new voices.

ARTHUR HIRSCH, UNITED STATES The Dana Alliance for Brain Initiatives, highly respected in Congress, has proclaimed that Parkinson's will likely be the first of the neurological diseases to be cured and that from the cure for Parkinson's they will develop the cures for other neurological diseases—possibly including Alzheimer's, Huntington's, and many others. If there be no other reason, this alone is reason enough to fully fund Parkinson's research as enacted into law as a part of the Udall Bill.

It would be unwise to ask that the money be spent unless we know that there are productive places to put it. But indeed, many there are! The theme for PAN's Public Policy Forum this year (1999) was "Raising Our Voices for a Cure." Several years ago, that might have seemed overoptimistic. But then again, the relief being provided to many through DBS (deep brain stimulation) might also have sounded like so much fiction not very long ago.

Scientists hold a lot of hope for stem-cell research to provide one possible cure. Other cures are being pursued, too.... Substantial strides are being made in this direction, as well as in easing the pain and slowing the progress of the disease.

(See Chapter 8 for more about promising Parkinson's research.)

JIM CORDY I couldn't help but think back to when the Udall Bill was introduced several years ago, when Congressman Upton said, "We can cure Parkinson's for the price of an on-ramp on an interstate."

HILARY BLUE, SOUTH AFRICA/ISRAEL/VIRGINIA If I managed to see my congressman, so can you. You don't have to be somebody special or famous; you just have to be yourself, and be persistent and polite!

I am a widow, 49 years old, with three teenage children. I was diagnosed with PD 16 years ago, when I was pregnant with my second child—but I'd had symptoms for many years before that. My friend Anne was diagnosed just 6 months ago.

We decided to attend the 1999 PAN Forum in D.C., and we frantically started collecting signatures for a petition to our congressman. We linked up with Sue, a veteran in PD advocacy, who lives in the same congressional district as we do, and who became our mentor.

Then last week I found out that our representative would be addressing a meeting at a local community center. I thought this would be an ideal opportunity to present our petition—little did I know how near perfect it would turn out to be.

Some at the meeting were woefully ignorant about PD. Anne reminded our congressman of when her son was his paper boy and then thanked him personally "on behalf of his loyal constituents" for his support of the Udall Bill—and she elicited from him a response that he would continue to support Parkinson's research, in particular the funding of the Udall Bill.

But the importance of the evening was not that we collared one congressman and presented him with a petition. I think we broke new ground—and fertile ground at that. We sparked an interest in a group of people who have now discovered a new interest, a new vulnerability. After all, any one of them may get PD. We did it. Anne and I. Two naive amateurs.

JEANETTE FUHR, MISSOURI It was reading posts about Ivan Suzman's interview on a Maine talk show that was the first seed implanted in my brain that perhaps I could be an advocate for Parkinson's. At that time, as a newly diagnosed PWP, I knew so little about the disease or what long-term life with PD could be about. So I learned, lurked, and eventually participated.

Now, I, too, am an advocate and I feel proud that my senator has taken the step with the other ten senators to address the issue of the Udall Act being carried out as originally stated.

As a community, we PWPs and our friends, families, and concerned other persons must keep reminding those who represent us in D.C. that we are watching and observing what is promised and what is actually done. We have to be informed and keep informing others of the need for Parkinson's research.

Partnerships to Cure Parkinson's

As the Parkinson's advocacy movement acquired recognition and increased funding for research, many activists came to recognize the importance of collaboration between all those involved in the search for a cure and improved care for PWP. The importance of cooperative efforts among Parkinson's patients, caregivers, PD organizations, government agencies, political leaders, and other health-advocacy groups continues. These are a few prime examples of the power of community:

Parkinson's Unity Walk

One of the first groups to encourage all PD organizations to work cooperatively, the Parkinson's Unity Walk is a fund-raising event that takes place in New York City each fall. Founded by Margot Zobel and Ken Aidekman and run by volunteers, the group's mission is to: (1) increase public awareness and understanding of Parkinson's disease; (2) promote unity within the Parkinson's community; and (3) raise funds for the ongoing research and study of Parkinson's disease, with the goal of discovering a cure or better treatment.

The Walk began in 1994 with 200 participants. At the 2000 Walk, an estimated 5,000 people joined together in Central Park, and over $600,000 was raised, to be divided among four major Parkinson's organizations. (See the resource guide for more information about the Unity Walk.)

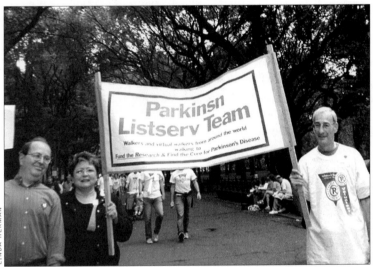

(From left) Ed Herman, Barbara Schirloff, and Mark Schirloff representing the Parkinsn listserv at the 2000 Unity Walk in New York City

JOHN TESTA, NEW YORK This year was our third time at the Unity Walk. We totally agree with the emphasis on unity. There were over 5,000 people who came from all over to be a part of this gathering of "family." I saw people who came with assorted types of canes and wheelchairs, people who with the physical support of others walked proudly in the Unity Walk.

Another great experience was getting to meet a lot of you from the Parkinson's list, whom we have only known through your postings.

The Parkinson's Alliance: Funding Promising Research

The Parkinson's Alliance is a nonprofit fund-raising organization whose sole mission is to raise money for the best Parkinson's researchers doing the most promising research. Currently led by Margaret and Martin Tuchman, Carol Walton, and Jim Maurer, the alliance conducts fund-raising events across the United States. Through their many partnerships and matching-fund affiliations within the Parkinson's community, they guarantee that for every dollar donated, two dollars will go directly to Parkinson's disease research.

In 2000, the alliance helped fund 43 pilot-study programs for a total of $2.4 million. They are committed to helping the NIH realize its goal of finding a cure by 2005. (See the resource guide, appendix 2, for more information.)

Fostering Patient Involvement in Research in the European Community

DIETMAR WESSEL EUROPARK joined a research consortium of companies from the UK, Greece, and Italy that received funding from the European Commission for the development of a viable tele-medicine product and assistive technology for the enhancement of motor performances in Parkinson's disease. The project PARREHA (Parkinsonian's Rehabilitation) will use virtual reality and auditory feedback in a computer-based system. The project is expected to last until the end of 2002. [I am] the patients' representative in the consortium.

FDA-Patient Initiative in the United States:

PERRY COHEN, WASHINGTON, D.C. Relations were also established with the Agency for Healthcare Research and Quality, which began an evidence-based review for PD at the suggestion of the House Appropriations Committee. Late in 2000, the crucial role of the FDA and the pharmaceutical industry in creating safe and effective treatments was acknowledged, and a program was initiated to incorporate the voices of patients in the design of clinical trials for drug evaluation.

Ad Hoc Coordinating Group Promotes Unity with NIH

PERRY COHEN While the national PD organizations each have ongoing relations with National Institutes of Health (NIH), particularly with the National Institute of Neurological Disease and Stroke (NINDS), they began working together early in 1999 in an ad hoc Washington coordination group. In the process, a working relationship was established on behalf of the collective PD community with Dr. Gerald Fischbach, director of the NINDS. A similar working relationship was established with the director of National Institute of Environmental Health Science (NIEHS), Dr. Ken Olden, who was planning a major program on investigating environmental causes of PD. Other important relations have been established with the Centers for Disease Control, particularly the National Center for Health Statistics.

More unified than ever before, the PD community focused first on research funding, and subsequently on the development of a public-private partnership to cure PD and on the development of a neurodegenerative initiative at NIH.

JIM CORDY Absolutely incredible! That's the only way I can describe the daylong meeting we had with a cross section of directors of the National Institutes of Health (NIH). They were interested, attentive, innovative, sympathetic, and, above all, committed to helping cure Parkinson's *now*. I believe we have embarked upon a partnership with NIH, and NINDS in particular, that will cure Parkinson's. That has always been our dream, and words cannot adequately describe the emotions I felt as I actually witnessed the pieces of the foundation put into place. It appears to be a real, solid foundation.

We have battled so long and so hard. We have accomplished what was thought to be impossible—passing the Morris K. Udall Bill—only to find out that effort was insufficient to turn the money spigot on. And far too often, we found ourselves portrayed as adversaries with NIH because of the earmarking issue. I stated earlier this year that it was time to be partners with NIH in curing this sinister disease. Never did I dream we would ever attain the atmosphere of commitment and cooperation that we saw.

A Blueprint for Curing Parkinson's

The following are excerpts from the National Institutes of Health's *Parkinson's Disease Research Agenda 2000–2005*:

A new optimism that Parkinson's disease can be defeated is energizing the research community and patient advocates. Halting the progression of Parkinson's disease, restoring lost function, and even preventing the disease are all realistic goals. This hope is fueled by the accelerating pace of discovery in neuroscience research generally, by advances in understanding what causes Parkinson's disease, and by a wide range of new treatments on the horizon, including stem cell transplants, precision surgical repair, chronic brain stimulation, and natural growth factors, to name a few....

While this document is properly focused on Parkinson's disease research, the relevance of this research agenda for other diseases should be noted. Parkinson's disease research can lead the way in the fight against all forms of neurodegeneration. The converse is also true. Research on other types of neurodegeneration may provide vital clues to curing Parkinson's disease....

Representatives from several Parkinson's advocacy groups were actively engaged in the planning process leading to this report. NIH found their involvement exceedingly useful and constructive. NIH is committed to working collaboratively with the Parkinson's community to refine and update the Parkinson's Disease Research Agenda, to implement the agenda to the extent funding permits, and to monitor its progress.[6]

PERRY COHEN I have read the draft NIH plan, and I am quite excited about the real commitment to PD research that the plan represents.

I do not think our work is done yet, however. We still need all the "wonderful PD advocates" (as Gerry Fischbach described me when he introduced me to his wife) who speak out to their elected officials. The political support that you and I and every one of our increasingly powerful grassroots advocates provide is essential to assure continued federal funding for PD. The ideas and concerns we provide are also critical to assure that the funding is directed toward new knowledge *and* to translating knowledge into delivery of effective treatments to the population.

A New Voice Brings New Visibility to PD Advocacy

> What celebrity has given me is the opportunity to raise the visibility of Parkinson's disease and focus more attention on the desperate need for more research dollars.
>
> MICHAEL J. FOX[7]

In May 2000, actor Michael J. Fox quit his popular and successful television series to devote full-time attention to Parkinson's advocacy. The newly created Michael J. Fox Foundation for Parkinson's Research awarded four grants within a few weeks, and fifteen additional grants totaling $1.5 million were awarded in April 2001. The Foundation joined with the Parkinson's Action Network for the 2000 Public Policy Forum. It was attended by over 200 advocates from all over the country, who returned home informed, energized, and inspired to organize their local Parkinson's communities to be "Invisible No More."

The Fruits of Grassroots Advocacy

In the 9 years since Joan Samuelson and Anne Udall first walked the halls of Capitol Hill, thousands of others have joined them, and as a result:

- ▸ Eleven new Udall Parkinson's Research Centers have been funded by the NIH.
- ▸ In February 2001, the Department of Veteran's Affairs announced funding for six additional PD centers focusing on research, education, and clinical care.
- ▸ Cooperative efforts are taking place between the National Institutes of Health, Congress, Parkinson's organizations, and people with Parkinson's.
- ▸ A bipartisan congressional working group on Parkinson's disease has been established.

▸ There has been increased funding for focused Parkinson's research and for the NIH as a whole, recognizing the crucial need to provide adequate funds for all medical research.

▸ The Parkinson's community has gained visibility.

▸ Many PWPs have become personally empowered by getting involved in the political process and learning that they can make a difference.

Team Parkinson

JIM CORDY   It is growing; it is gaining momentum. I first sensed its presence many years ago when Joan Samuelson spoke the words "invisible no more" to an eclectic group of ragtag advocates.... Michael J. Fox has given it unimaginable visibility. Mary Yost epitomized its resolve and persistence as she crossed the finish line of last year's L.A. marathon wearing the Team Parkinson jersey.

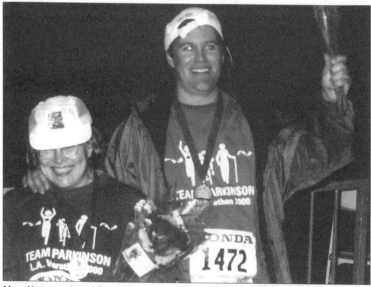

Mary Yost, member of Team Parkinson, at the 2000 L.A. Marathon

Team Parkinson is more than an entry in a walk or race. It is that power we feel when we join together. Those fortunate enough to have gone to a Public Policy Forum, a Unity Walk, or the L.A. Marathon have felt its power. We have seen what can be accomplished if we all pull together toward a common goal: the thought-to-be-impossible passing of the Udall Bill.

Team Parkinson is a group, a spirit that willingly places the goal of curing PD ahead of individual goals. It is the banner under which all who battle this disease may rally. It is the researchers, the advocates, the politicians, and the people with Parkinson's. It is an elite team with only one requirement for participation: the pledge to put curing PD as the first priority.

Endnote: "Thanks, Mo!"

Mo Udall died on 12 December 1998, at the age of 76, his long struggle with Parkinson's disease finally over.

KEN AIDEKMAN For most, Mo Udall will be remembered as the congressman from the state of Arizona with the marvelous sense of humor: a striking, determined figure who championed environmental causes, stood up for the rights of the common man, and all the while maintained his honor, setting the highest standards of bipartisanship, fairness, and good will. But for people with Parkinson's and their loved ones, Mo Udall's legacy will forever include a piece of legislation that he did not write or nurture through Congress: The Morris K. Udall Parkinson's Research and Education Act. Even after his retirement from public office, his enduring good name did much to bring about a brighter future for millions of Americans.

Many people worked long and hard to pass the Udall Bill. At times, it seemed as if the battle would be lost. But just at the lowest point, a former colleague might mention the great esteem he or she held for Mo. Or maybe a legislative aide would recount a joke or clever story he or she had once heard him tell. We began to understand the depth of love that remained for Mo Udall in our nation's capital years after his public service had ended.

We may not have known Mo personally, but his presence was palpable. As we learned more and more about his accomplishments and strength of character, his persona became a rallying point. He put a familiar face on our common cause. We implored others to "Do it for Mo." We began to look on him with the pride one feels for a hometown friend who has made good. He was more than just a well-known congressman with PD. Mo's reputation was such that, whatever the contents of the bill, it was important to work on it because his name was attached to it.

Perhaps it is unfair to forever link the Udall name with Parkinson's. After all, Mo's life was much more than the malady he fought for two decades. But for the Parkinson's community, the Mo Udall Act has come to represent something greater than a simple act to authorize spending. It stands for our hard-learned education in the practical use of political action to accomplish just goals. These goals included getting our elected representatives to recognize the immense problem Parkinson's poses for America and convincing them to dedicate a fair share of our nation's resources to finding a cure. Surely, Mo would not object to the association of his name with a noble cause such as this.

Thanks, Mo!

chapter 7

When Drugs Fail: Surgeries for Parkinson's Disease

D RUG THERAPY PROVIDES satisfactory relief from Parkinson's symptoms for a number of years for most PD patients. However, eventually, as the dopamine level in the brain continues to fall, medication side effects begin to outweigh the benefits. Dyskinesia, that is, uncontrollable excessive movement, is a very common side effect of long-term use of levodopa, and it can become more disabling than PD symptoms themselves. A study of young-onset PD patients found that after five years of levodopa treatment, 91 percent experienced dyskinesia; after 10 years, it affected virtually 100 percent of the subjects.[1]

In addition, a wearing-off effect may occur—the medication becomes less effective and works for shorter periods, and doses must be increased and taken more frequently. Off periods become more frequent and disabling. When various combinations of medications no longer control symptoms adequately, or unacceptable side effects develop, surgical options may be considered.

Three types of Parkinson's surgeries are currently being performed or are under investigation: lesioning surgery (pallidotomy), deep brain stimulation (DBS), and cell transplantation.

Pallidotomy

Pallidotomy is a neurosurgical lesioning procedure that involves insertion of an electrode probe into the globus pallidus, destroying neurons in this region of the brain, which have become overactive in patients with Parkinson's disease.

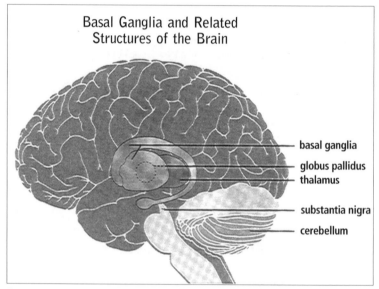

Target areas of the brain for PD treatments (From FDA Consumer article by John Henkel. "Parkinson's Disease: New Treatments Slow Onslaught of Symptoms." (July–August 1998), p. 17.)

In order to provide the surgeon with required feedback, the patient must be awake throughout the operation. Improvements in stereotactic imaging techniques now allow surgeons to more accurately position the probe, but there are still risks of complications. Stroke is the most serious, occurring in about 1 percent to 3 percent of cases.

The damage caused to targeted brain cells during a pallidotomy is permanent; however, it may bring substantial improvement in the quality of life for certain patients, by relieving tremor, rigidity, bradykinesia (slow movement), and dyskinesia.

A New Member of the "Hole-in-the-Head Gang"

Kees Paap has lived with PD for over 10 years. His symptoms became extremely disabling, as he described in Chapter 2, and he underwent a pallidotomy in June 1999. Kees shared with the PIEN the following accounts of his decision-making process, surgical experiences, and results:

May 10, 1999

Hi list friends,
My quality of life has been good till the beginning of this year. It became worse, and finally it got bad enough to go for surgery.

What do I think about the surgery? People have asked me that many times. I'd rather *not* think about it. I know what will happen and I know the risks, but I am "ready" for it. Faye answers to the same question that she is scared, but she also knows I am "ready" for it. So we are thinking a lot about it. We have talked a lot about it and we both know how the surgery is done. I hope Faye can be with me in the operating room so she can support me and help me when my English is failing me because of the tension or from other causes. I would like her to be with me as my wife and not as a surgeon, although she probably will see it from both sides.

I will keep you informed about my experiences.

May 26

We went full of optimism to Dallas. When I came in, I was very off; when it was my turn, I was very good. But fortunately I got dyskinetic before I was through. I say "fortunately" because I was afraid I was not going to be treated at all. Two doctors independent from each other made the conclusion that I was a very good candidate for a pallidotomy because of the following reasons:

1. I am a young patient.
2. I am healthy.
3. I am mentally healthy.
4. I have Parkinson's on one side.
5. I am not having tremors.
6. I don't have blockades.
7. I have a good response on levodopa.

So, seven good reasons why I should go for the pallidotomy. I was not quite sure yet—the pallidotomy is irreversible—but after some talking, I was convinced that this was the best for me. Certainly I felt more convinced after a few details were better explained. The most important one was the way they wanted to do it. They have a physiologist who makes the calculations with the help of very fine computer equipment. This method is called micro-electrode recording (MER). I don't know exactly how it works but it is a method with sounds, a probe, a computer, and three experts. So I said yes.

June 5

I didn't sleep. I stayed awake all night. Faye slept for an hour. We left the house at 3:00 A.M. and arrived a little before 5:00 A.M. at the Presbyterian Hospital in Dallas. X rays and blood tests were already done in Waco.

We went through the process of administration, and at 7:15 they were ready to place the "crown." The crown is screwed in the head with four screws. This hurts a little, but I was willing to accept a whole lot more pain to get rid of my PD symptoms. I was rolled through a few long gangways to the OR. I felt like a robot man that could think but not move. I was at that moment very off, and about the only thing I could move were my eyes, looking through the bars of the crown. An MRI was made with the crown on.

I was lucky enough to have the newest operating table, which is very comfortable for the back. I was introduced to everyone in the OR. First my head (the crown) was fixed on the special connector. I was wrapped in several layers of plastic and sheets and was not supposed to see anything. I relaxed as well as possible and chatted a little with the head nurse. Everyone was very friendly. I appreciated that they explained everything they did. Then the drilling of the hole started. This and the breaking of the skull was the worst thing, but by far not as bad as I anticipated.

So the procedure began. The probe went a little deeper. They kept on trying it until they were both (the neurologist and the technician for the MER method) satisfied. Then they started sending pulses through it, activating the probe as a stimulator. I started counting from one to 20 and backwards. Nothing happened. A little more activity. A slight tingling in the fingers. Not a good result. The probe went a little deeper. Counting till my voice started trembling. A little more. My arm went straight up into a cramp. I couldn't speak! A very nasty experience. Of course, they saw it very fast, because they watched me carefully.

The probe came all the way out and was injected under a slightly different angle. Amazing results!! I could tap my hand!! Make the bird's beak open and close!! The probe was replaced by a device that formed the lesions. Two lesions were made. At a little past noon, I was parked in the recovery room. But I was way too good for that. Pretty soon I was taken to another room, where I finally could sleep for a while. In the evening, they let me hang my legs out of the bed. And after a good night's rest, I dressed myself and was walking around. I was scanned at 1:00 P.M., and then I got to go home.

I went home as a new *human being*. You can believe me when I tell you that I cried from happiness. It was such a difference!!

June 6

Dear friends,
It is Saturday morning, almost 24 hours after the surgery. I want to describe what my feelings are. I feel so grateful to our Lord, who made all this possible. Also, I am grateful to my surgeon and the staff of surgeons, nurses, and helpers who were present at the surgery. I am so truly grateful for my wonderful recovery. It is amazing how many people have been praying for me. It is just wonderful that these people were not disappointed. I am feeling wonderful; I really do. The fact that I can type this so easily is a sign that I am doing much better. Very grateful I am to Faye, who has been a tigress for me. She watched over me as if I was her cub. And actually, I felt like I was. But now I will be her husband again. I will be active again. I have been not very active lately. Not only physically but also mentally very tired. That is all over now. I feel refreshed. I will need a week to recover, but then I will be great and I will pick up all the things I let go. I will clean our house, do the garden, and many other things. I am so full of my old energy again.

June 7

I feel great. Slept very well, and I went to church to thank everyone for their prayers. I am very well and I am not tired at all. My head is all short hair and a shaved spot. I have ten "staples" in my head. My private doctor will remove them.

June 8

I played table tennis last night. I also went to the driving range. Tonight I go bowling.

June 15

Tomorrow our trip to New York starts. So today Faye removes the staples. The wound is closing very nicely. My shaved head grows hair again.

June 26

I feel like I did seven or eight years ago. I am still experimenting with medicines. I can take less but am not sure how much less. I have no dyskinesia. I go off very slowly and never so far anymore. I am healthy!!! Well, almost. I hope it stays this way. My toes are cramping sometimes. I still have little problems, but I am ready for the fight again.

I love you all.

October 29, 1999

I am busy with my bowling event this weekend. I will bowl 28 hours for funding of the search for the cause and the cure. The world record I will try to break is to bowl 52,000 points in 24 hours. That is, 300 games with an average of 175 pins. It will be very difficult, but I am going for it!

More Young Members

Joan Snyder was diagnosed in 1991, at age 39, and underwent pallidotomy surgery in 1996. She wrote:

I can't run a Boston marathon, but I can go to a meeting and push my cart in the grocery store. My daughter, Ali, says that Dr. Henderson put yeses into her mother's brain. "She used to say no, we couldn't go places and I couldn't have friends over to spend the night—but now she says yes."

Barb Mallut's pallidotomy took place in 1994, 12 years after her diagnosis at age 40. She had experienced undiagnosed symptoms for at least 8 years prior to her diagnosis. She wrote:

1997

Yesterday was the third anniversary—or, as I call it, my "rebirth-day"—of my unilateral pallidotomy. To this day, I'm *so* thankful for having had the surgery. The surgery was performed on the left side of my brain to relieve PD symptoms on the right side of my body. Beneficial results were immediate. Today, my right side remains exactly as it was after the surgery—*externally*, there are no visible Parkinson's signs at all (right side only). There has been no visible diminishment of the benefits I received from the surgery.

The disease has since moved into the left side of my body, and there are whole-inner-body symptoms and sensations on both sides (i.e., both vocal cords are involved). I am troubled by profound daily fatigue.

While I get angry and frustrated by the PD symptoms as they develop on my left side, the pallidotomy seems to have got rid of the "Barb-imitating-a-slab-of-wood" look and feeling that I had prior to the surgery.

1999

I've regained full movement in my right side—arm, hand, fingers, leg, and foot feel totally and remain "normal." Internally, things still continue to degenerate, though I have no idea if such degeneration was slowed down initially by the surgery or exacerbated by it.

While the right side continues to function well, the left side is now manifesting symptoms, though there's a marked difference between the external symptoms I had with my right side and those I now have on the left side. It could be almost a different disease if one went by the symptoms I now experience.

I'll be forever grateful for that pallidotomy because it was like being given a second chance at life. However, I probably will not have another pallidotomy, as in my case, I feel deep brain stimulation would be of more benefit.

Update 2000

So far (knocking on wood), my right side still remains for all intents and purposes "normal." The left side, after initially showing up with some symptoms, seems to have settled down, reminding me that it's there with an occasional "resting tremor."

I also have a little tremoring in my jaw periodically—aggravating, but nothing I can't handle.

Pallidotomy isn't a cure, but for me, it gave me the feeling that I was back in the human race.

Deep Brain Stimulation (DBS)

The last decade has lead to a true renaissance in surgical approaches for Parkinson's disease. This was the direct result of the powerful model for Parkinson's disease, which has allowed us to learn a great deal about the circuitry of the basal ganglia. For the first time we know where to intervene to balance out the abnormal brain circuits in Parkinson's disease. A particularly exciting innovation is the use of deep brain stimulation. DR. WILLIAM LANGSTON, PARKINSON'S INSTITUTE, CALIFORNIA[2]

Deep brain stimulation (DBS) is a surgical therapy in which an electrode is implanted into a target site in the brain—currently the thalamus, globus pallidus, or subthalamus. The electrode is then connected under the skin to a pulse generator (similar to a pacemaker) that is implanted under the collarbone. High-frequency stimulation from the electrode blocks neuronal activity, having a similar effect as a pallidotomy lesion. However, the stimulation techniques are reversible and do not cause damage to the brain. The stimulation can be turned on and off with the use of a handheld magnet placed over the generator.

DBS of the Thalamus

The thalamus was the first brain site studied for DBS, and stimulation of this area has been shown to be effective in treating tremor but is not beneficial for other PD symptoms, such as rigidity or slowness. Deep brain stimulation of the thalamus (Vim DBS) received FDA approval for treatment of tremor in 1997.

DBS of the Globus Pallidus

Preliminary data suggests that electrical stimulation of the globus pallidus (GPi DBS) reduces tremor, levodopa-induced dyskinesia (involuntary movements), bradykinesia (slowness), and rigidity.[3] This procedure is considered experimental in the United States and as of February 2001 had not yet received FDA approval.

DBS of the Subthalamic Nucleus

The most recent studies of electrode implantation in the subthalamic nucleus (STN DBS) have been especially encouraging—resulting in substantial reductions in tremor, slowness, and rigidity, *and* the lowering of levodopa dosages. Some patients reported being able to completely eliminate medication after DBS surgery. STN DBS has been routinely performed in Europe for a number of years, also with promising results. In March 2000, an FDA advisory committee recommended approval for deep brain stimulation to treat the four major motor symptoms of Parkinson's disease. Full FDA approval was still pending as of June 2001.

Research continues to better understand how deep brain stimulation works and to identify the optimal implantation site for each patient. Following are accounts by PIEN list members who were among the pioneers of DBS surgery.

On 18 May 1999, in Chicago, PIEN member Dr. Charlie Meyer underwent surgery for deep brain stimulation of the subthalamic nucleus area of the brain, one of the newest and most promising surgical treatments for advanced Parkinson's disease. Another list member, Jane Ross of Oregon, was a volunteer subject in one of the first experimental studies of DBS techniques in the United States, initiated in 1996 at the Oregon Health Sciences University.

28 May 1999
From: Charlie Meyer

After getting out of bed and into my wheelchair as usual, I went to the computer and read my mail and composed the response below. Then I decided to get up and try to walk, which I did with my walker with amazing ease. My wife was incredulous. You have to realize that even transfers were extremely difficult. I went downstairs for the first time in a year to wake up my son. I took a shower, then called my mother, who was in tears, chilled a bottle of champagne, and walked around again. Truly amazing! Still some adjustments to be made, but I'm on my way!!! STN (subthalamic nucleus) DBS is clearly the wave of the future—at least for me. It is truly a miraculous change, even on the first adjustment.

29 May 1999
From: Jane Ross

Charles,
You will never know how happy I am for you. I guess I can start breathing in and out again. I have been holding my breath until the other shoe hit the floor, and it sounds like it is off and running. While you improve, I predict that you will feel better each day until there will be days that you actually forget you have Parkinson's. I wish you well!

29 May 1999
From: Charlie Meyer

Jane,
And you will never know how happy I am for your having benefited from this wonderful procedure for the last 3 years and how grateful I am to you for pioneering this work.

A Personal Account

Jane Ross was diagnosed with PD in 1979, at the age of 37. She wrote the following about her surgery:

JANE ROSS, OREGON My husband and I have been living with my Parkinson's disease for almost twenty years. It was Halloween

1979, when I depended on a CAT scan to tell me if my tremors were from a brain tumor or from Parkinson's disease. I remember the nurse saying, "Let's hope for Parkinson's." Well, I got my wish that day. I was young, 37; I could handle it....

It wasn't until about seven years later, in 1986, that my tremors multiplied to the other side. It then became a full time job taking care of myself and my family.

Making the Decision

In 1992, when time-released levodopa was first put on the market, I tried it and developed dyskinesia because it was too strong. After doing that, I never was able to use levodopa again without the ugly extra movements. I went downhill. Which was worse, the dyskinesia or the tremors? I chose tremors, but that left me unable to do much of anything. I had become a victim of Parkinson's disease.

In October 1995, I went for my regular neurological checkup and my doctor said, "There isn't anything else I can do for you. Would you consider an operation?" I said I was willing to find out if they could help me. So appointments were made in Portland to...see [a neurosurgeon] to discuss pallidotomy.

At that time in Portland, Oregon, something new and exciting was taking place. The Oregon Health Sciences University was planning a new research project, called deep brain stimulation. Within the next year, they were planning to do ten experimental surgeries on volunteers, with the stimulators being placed in one or the other of two brain locations, the thalamus or the pallidum. Part of the protocol was that it would be a "blind" study (that is, I wasn't to be told in which location my stimulator was placed). I am still "blinded" in regard to this aspect....

DBS Is Reversible

My reasons for having deep brain stimulation instead of a pallidotomy were twofold. I was impressed that the DBS would be "reversible," and since I was only 54 years old at that time, there still might be a cure in my lifetime.

The other reason was that even though there was a possibility that the procedure would leave me unable to speak while the stimulator was turned on, I would be able to turn it off in order to regain my speaking ability.

The most personal reason was so my husband could still turn me on!...

"I Remember Only the Good Parts"

The operation lasted five and a half hours; fortunately, I don't remember most of it. It was kind of like having a baby in that I only remember the good parts.

I try to forget that my blood pressure went way over 200 and that it was extremely painful to have the "halo" screwed into my skull. I try to forget that I wet the bed when they left me alone for too long right after the surgery. My head was shaved and one thing I wasn't prepared for was the swelling around my eyes with a yellow fluid-like substance.

I remember the moment my left hand quit trembling and my right hand too, almost, and I remember crying uncontrollably after it was all over.

I had a week in the hospital to wait for the second part of the operation—the implanting of the pacemaker controls on both sides. I painted my fingernails during my free time, a luxury I hadn't been able to indulge for years.

Benefits and Side Effects

During that week they came each day and tried different settings on the computerized pacemakers. Each time they changed the settings, I got an electrical shock in my right leg strong enough to lift my leg off the bed and render me speechless. Needless to say, I could have done without that!

Another immediate result of the surgery showed up as soon as I got into a car. Before the surgery, as a front-seat passenger, I frequently had the illusion that other vehicles were coming at us in our car, and I would dodge and flail in self-defense (very disturbing to the driver!). That's gone, thank God!

Some changes were unexpected, like my new need for nine hours of sleep, instead of the former four hours. My body temperature came back down to normal, and I suffered no more hot flashes. Other side effects were less welcome, like the "lightning" out of the corner of my eye every once in a while, or the constant distortion and cramping of my left foot, or my slurred speech.

The surgery was really scary. Although I wouldn't want to do it again, I still feel it was worth the results. The benefits in terms of my Parkinson's symptoms were dramatic. Two years later, my tremor is still gone on the left side, and my right side is much improved.

I am still learning to balance the time on and off to get maximum benefits, i.e., how long to turn the stimulator off before I get the full effects back. If I leave it on more than three days, the improvement on my right side wanes; it feels like it isn't turned on at all. Right now it seems to work best if I turn it off overnight.

Costs Are a Major Factor

One of the most common questions I get is about the cost. People need to know that not all health insurance companies will cover this procedure (as of 1999). Our insurance company let us down; after the surgery, they decided not to pay for it. Their decision left us with an enormous debt; the doctor's bill was $5,000; the hospital's was $16,000; and the hardware was $12,000; resulting in a grand total of $33,000. When the batteries run down, the whole unit will need to be replaced at a cost of an additional $12,000 or more.

We have finally finished paying for it; I may never get a new diamond, or get to take a cruise, but I'm just happy to be alive and doing so well with Parkinson's disease.[4]

Update: Early 2000

My surgery will be 4 years old in March.... Others who (had DBS) surgery are still taking levodopa. I am not. There are only 10 of us in the study and I have only met one of them and he isn't doing as well as I am. I don't mean to brag but be truthful. I no longer see lightning out the corner of my eye but still have the other side effects, cramping in the left foot and slowed speech rather than slurred speech.

I turn the stimulator off overnight and it seems fine in the morning. When I had the battery replaced last fall, they changed the setting.... I really should go back for a "fine tuning," but it is 300 miles to the office, and this setting is okay, but not as good as the one I had before the battery change....

I am sorry to say, I haven't met anyone [who] is doing as well as I am. It would be hard to tell unless you saw the before and after view.

Update: September 2000

First, I am doing very well and I think I have improved as much as I will. Most of my improvement was during the third year after the operation. It truly has been a heavenly change in my life. But I'm not convinced that this is the answer to a cure. It has too many variables. And it is life-risking surgery.

Since surgery, I have been dependent on my surgeon for appointments, and he is 300 miles away. This year I have been back twice for an adjustment and a consultation.... He is the only one doing adjustments in Oregon. It is important to realize that after the surgery, the patient is still committed to the surgeon or staff for the rest of their life.

Another View: Dick Swindler's DBS of the Globus Pallidus

Dick and Marge Swindler are from Kansas. In 1995, Dick was 51 and had had Parkinson's for 14 years when he became one of the first Americans to undergo surgery to implant electrodes into the globus pallidus area of his brain, at Kansas University Medical Center.

Why Dick Volunteered for Experimental DBS Surgery

DICK I chose pallidal stimulation because of the reversibility of the procedure. If a new procedure comes up in the future, I wanted my brain intact so it could be performed. In a regular pallidotomy, a scar is left on the brain that can't be removed. This could affect the results of a newer surgery. My pre-op symptoms consisted of a strong tremor, severe dystonia in my feet, and some dyskinesia, and the levodopa was becoming less effective than it had been.

MARGE Prior to the surgery, he had had to go on disability from his job as a high school math teacher of 28 years. He had severe tremor in his left arm and right leg, plus a bit of dyskinesia and a great deal of painful dystonia. He was taking a relatively small amount of levodopa, etc., but couldn't tolerate any more because of the severity of the dystonia and additional dyskinesia. He had progressed to having *no* good "on" times—he was "off" a good part of the time, and the remainder of the time was "on" with dystonia. That was what made him a candidate for this experimental surgery. (He was the third in the United States to have it done.)

Encouraging Early Results

DICK Following the operation, I lost most of the tremor and dystonia. Also, the levodopa has become effective again. My most disturbing symptom was the tremor. I now have control of it about 90 percent of the time.

Update: 2000

MARGE Dick had 4 excellent years postsurgery before needing to have his stimulator settings increased. He has now been diagnosed with PD for nearly 19 years. This year his PD has seemingly begun progressing more rapidly, so he has had three stimulator-setting increases, counting the one last December. The good news is that so far, new settings have taken care of the increased symptoms. He is almost 5 years postsurgery now, and his batteries seem to be going strong.

I can't stress enough how greatly his quality of life improved after the surgery. He had been unable to do anything but sit in his chair and shake, and not only couldn't he hold a book, but he couldn't concentrate. His symptoms were greatly improved after the surgery and continued to improve for some time. By 1 year post-surgery, the little bit of residual tremor had disappeared, and the other symptoms seemed better, too.

The symptoms that showed up this year were freezing, balance problems, and when he was more "off," some cognitive and memory problems. His tremor still hasn't returned. We continue to be surprised and pleased that a few minor stimulator adjustments can "fix" the new symptoms as they appear. We don't know how long this will continue to be the case, but he is a long way from reaching the maximum settings on his stimulator, so there's considerable hope for the future.

GPi DBS, which I've referred to as pallidal stimulation, is no longer the surgery of choice, since STN DBS is considered to control a wider variety of symptoms. Nevertheless, the gross motor symptoms plus cognitive deficits seem to be greatly improved by his GPi. We're grateful to Dr. Wilkinson and Dr. William Koller for what amounted to nearly a life-saving surgery.

STN DBS

The subthalamic nucleus (STN) is currently considered the optimal surgery site for many patients, since it improves all of the major symptoms of PD—tremor, rigidity, bradykinesia, and dyskinesia. Dr. William Langston of the Parkinson's Institute states, "Indications are that between ten to thirty per cent of patients may be able to go entirely off medications. But to continue this work, a great deal of work needs to be done, both experimentally and in practice. We still don't understand how it works and we may not have found the best area to stimulate yet."[5]

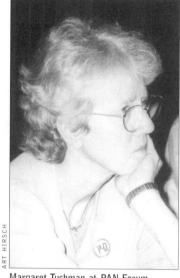

ART HIRSCH

Margaret Tuchman at PAN Forum

MARGARET TUCHMAN, NEW JERSEY I decided to have DBS at the end of last summer (2000); I had a long talk with husband and friends and we agreed that this was a good temporary step to take until the cure is found.

I'd had enough of the unpredictability of meds. Dyskinesia during the day and my nightly bradykinesia, with the accompanying stutter steps were the enemy. I needed to feel better *now*!

On 28 December 2000, I had bilateral STN at NYU Medical Center. It is a fascinating experience! To be awake and hear all that goes around you during surgery and then to sit and be "tuned" by a person sitting at a computer playing with levels of voltage. It's pretty amazing!

My stimulator was turned on 2 weeks after surgery, and I've had seven adjustments since. Each adjustment has produced improvement—some minor, some significant. This is where one has to be patient and persevere. I know that STN has not cured my "debilitating progressive condition," but sometimes I find it hard to believe that I am not disease free. I no longer have dyskinesia or bradykinesia with the accompanying stutter steps. I haven't bumped into anything, nor fallen. I don't have the pain in my neck and shoulder. If I look into the mirror, I see a symmetrical face, my left eyelid does not droop, I can smile, my voice is okay, and I feel good. I am feeling better than I have felt since I can't remember when, and I am taking less medication.

My decision to have surgery came as a result of thorough research and fully understanding the procedure and the post-surgery adjustments. The neurophysiologist looked straight into my eyes during our presurgery visit and said, "Commit right now that you will always be careful and not jeopardize the stimulator or the surgery. If you are unwilling to take this very seriously, I don't want to waste time, energy, and money."

The surgical team should include experienced neurophysiologist(s) who participate in the surgery *and* provide the postoperative adjustments. The distance traveled to get ongoing follow-up is important, though quite a few STN patients fly in to New York to get their adjustments.

People considering DBS/STN should actually handle the battery-operated pulse generators and the stereotactic headgear. I thought the units were quite heavy, and the "halo" was something Hannibal Lecter should be wearing.

As soon as the FDA approves the use of the Medtronic stimulator and the battery-operated pulse generators for Parkinson's, we can look forward to technical improvements of the instrumentation. Some advancements are already in use in Europe. The one I am waiting for is being hooked up via phone and Internet to the doctor, so she/he can adjust the patient videophonically (my term).

PETER DAWKINS, AUSTRALIA My surgery was done to the subthalamic nucleus in 1997, and should not be confused with surgery to the globus pallidus, as this is an alternative site with very different results. The first thing to point out is that the results will really not be apparent for at least 3 months, as the voltage has to be adjusted and everyone is different. I am really only beginning to feel human again, and the bradykinesia or stiffness has gone.

I still take medication for the tremor in my legs, which is worse than before the surgery, but the medication has been reduced by half. I am by all accounts looking and feeling better, although I have my good days and bad days, but with none of the complications of before. Overall, I am still evaluating the results, and the jury is still out on the long-term benefits.

Update: October 2000

I had STN stimulation for Parkinson's 3½ years ago and have only recently had the program as near to perfect as it can be. It seems to vary a lot between patients and, of course, according to the progress of the PD. Just by sheer blind faith and fine-tuning my medication regime, I am now better than I have been since Parkinson came to call 12 years ago.

I accidentally turned one side off the other day and it was astounding. I had no hand tremor, only tremor in the legs at the time of the surgery, and now without the pacemakers it is quite apparent. It's not a cure for Parkinson's, but when done well, it provides incredible relief. I have cut my medications to ¼ of what they were.

Charlie Meyer: Update: November 2000

My surgery was 1½ years ago, and I am pleased with the results. Except for some dystonia in my right arm (the less-affected one), my symptoms are significantly reduced. I have no off periods at all, and I walk with a walker, where before I was wheelchair-bound. It takes time to adjust the IPG (pulse generators) correctly. Before the DBS, I took nine or ten Sinemet per day as well as one to three amantadine and 16–24 mg of Requip per day. Now I am down to 6 mg of Requip, ½ Sinemet, and 300 mg amatadine per day.

DBS: Summing Up

What are the benefits of DBS? Patients who are no longer helped by currently available medications eventually experience longer off times than on times, disabling dyskinesias, and increasing severity of other PD symptoms and levodopa side effects. DBS has been found to alleviate tremor, rigidity, bradykinesia, and dyskinesia. Most patients who have undergone DBS surgery report significant improvements in the quality of their lives for a number of years following the surgery. Compared to pallidotomy, the procedure is relatively nondestructive to brain tissue. It is adjustable and reversible, allowing patients to fully benefit from improved treatments or surgical techniques that may become available in the future.

However, there are potential complications and problems with DBS that must also be considered. There are surgical risks, especially bleeding in the brain, that could lead to a stroke (reported in 2 to 4 percent of patients). Infection from the stimulator hardware occurs in about 4 to 5 percent of patients. Ongoing stimulator adjustments are required to optimize treatment, and the battery must be replaced every 2 to 5 years. The equipment is very expensive, estimated at $10,000 per side in the United States (as of 1999), and not all health insurance will cover the surgical or follow-up expenses. It may be difficult to locate qualified, experienced neurosurgeons who are trained in this very specialized and exacting surgery, especially for those located far from large cities and medical centers. Further research is needed to determine the long-term effects of DBS and the optimal target site for each patient.

And, it is not a cure.

Fetal Cell Transplantation

When the 10-year ban on fetal-tissue research was lifted by President Bill Clinton in 1993, it reopened a route for scientific research that many believed could lead to a cure for PD and other degenerative diseases. Fetal cells rapidly divide and grow in new environments and are less likely to be rejected by the body's immune system than adult cells. Fetal brain cells can be transplanted to replace the dopamine-producing cells lacking in Parkinson's disease. A limited number of advanced-stage PD patients in the United States and other countries have been successfully treated with transplanted fetal cells, with benefits lasting 10 years or more for some individuals. Clinical trials utilizing fetal-pig brain cells are also underway, with promising preliminary results. This research has also helped advance new restorative techniques and therapies for PD and for other serious and life-threatening diseases. However, it has been surrounded by intense political, religious, and ethical debates.

To Denver with Hope: Lynda McKenzie's Story

Lynda McKenzie, a 46-year-old artist from Ontario, Canada, was diagnosed with Parkinson's disease in 1987. The disease progressed to the advanced stage, and Lynda was becoming increasingly disabled, unable even to get out of bed by herself. She was also suffering from severe dyskinesia and injuries from frequent falls. She took part in a 1996 clinical trial of fetal cell transplantation at the University of Colorado in Denver, knowing that according to the research protocol, she had a 50 percent chance of receiving an actual transplant and a 50 percent chance of receiving sham brain surgery.

Waiting for the Phone to Ring

After returning home from my last pre-op tests in New York, life became a waiting game. The phone call that would summon us to Denver for surgery would come on a Monday. Two days later, we would have to be on our way to the University of Denver, where the double-blind surgery would take place early Thursday morning. Each Monday I stayed close to home, jumping every time the phone gave its specially coded long-distance ring. Four Mondays passed that way. On the fifth, at just before 5:00 P.M., as I told myself all the good reasons why we would be waiting another week, the phone rang. Long distance. "Mrs. McKenzie? Your surgery is scheduled for this Thursday."

Thursday, University of Denver Hospital

"Good morning, Mrs. McKenzie. We're ready to start preparing you for surgery." Al came into my room and gave me a big hug. Behind him were Dr. Breeze and three nurses pushing a metal cart loaded with my halo, assorted hardware, needles, vials, and a Black and Decker drill.

Dr. Breeze introduced himself and explained calmly that the next few minutes would be the worst part of the whole procedure. Before I had a chance to dwell on that, they lowered the large medieval-looking stereotactic device (halo) over my head until the lower horizontal bars reached my nose. They then positioned the upper circular bar on my forehead. Dr. Breeze used a black magic marker to indicate the positions of the four screws that would hold the halo to my skull. Dr. Breeze filled several giant needles from a vial on the cart and dabbed a topical freezing solution on the four insertion points.

With one nurse holding my shoulders, another holding my head, and Al clutching my hands, Dr. Breeze inserted the first long needle into my forehead. The liquid burned. There's not a lot of flesh in that area, and he was right, it did hurt. Quickly he picked up a fresh needle and inserted it on the other side of my forehead. Two more needles in the back of my head and the halo was lowered into place. A few brackets were tightened so it fit as snugly as possible. Even though I had confidence in Dr. Breeze, the sight of his Black and Decker drill poised at my forehead was frightening.

"This tool does the best job I've found; the initial contact of the screw might hurt a bit, but when it gets past a certain area, it won't hurt any more." The nurses tightened their grips and he squeezed the power switch to "on." Initially, it felt like the sharp cut of a large knife, but it did ease up a bit. I heard the drill stop and start twice and felt his hand on the back of my head.

Then he positioned the drill over my right forehead and turned it on. This time the pain was incredible. I squeezed Al's hand and tears ran down my cheeks. I instinctively pulled back but the nurses held me, and all I could do was cry, "It hurts, it really, really hurts." It seemed an eternity before the drill stopped. Not realizing that the screws had already been inserted and tightened on the back, I remember thinking there was no way I could go through that pain again. If only there were a way to leap out of bed and run down the hall to *anywhere* else. Unfortunately, my traitor of a body was sufficiently cobbled by lack of medication and nurses that escaping wasn't an option.

The next challenge was to move my motionless body, complete with heavy metal cage, from bed to stretcher. Finally, propped with pillows under my neck, I was rolled out of the room past my roomie, Joy. She must have wondered what ancient form of torture had been going on behind the curtain.

As I rolled by her, I couldn't resist saying, "I bet you wish you had one of these too, eh, Joy!"

I was wheeled to the operating room. Nurses, technicians, surgeons were gowned and gloved. Everyone was ready for Dr. Breeze's arrival. While we waited, eyes peered down at me over green facemasks, and voices muffled by surgical masks introduced themselves.

"Hi, Lynda. I'm Sue. I'll be with you throughout the surgery."

"Don't worry, Lynda, you'll be up and moving soon."

"Hi, Lynda. I'm Frank. I'll be checking your blood pressure."

At that moment, I thought of a favorite joke of my dad's. It would be perfect for this moment! I couldn't let the opportunity go by. "Frank, now that we're in Denver, you know, near all those wonderful ski resorts, when this surgery is over, will I be able to ski?" Frank took my hand and quickly assured me that of course I would!

"Wow, that's great Frank! Because you know something, I never could get the hang of it before!"

Everyone in the room groaned; they'd been caught by one of the oldest jokes in the world! I contentedly rested on my laurels, thinking proudly how I'd aced the delivery of the joke even in my groggy state.

Suddenly, it was time to go into the operating room. Everyone sprang into action. The gurney began to move and Al kissed me. I was quickly wheeled into the operating room and transferred to a cold, hard table. Bolts held my halo to the table. I was totally immobile and immovable. I forced myself to keep awake and watch the activity in the room. All were focused on me and my failing brain. I focused on everyone who has Parkinson's now and everyone who will be diagnosed with it before the cause and cure are finally found. The bustling, blurry movement around me was almost dreamlike.

Finally. A year of medical questionnaires, videos, grueling tests, tears, and hopes. I firmly believed that within the hour the fetal tissue would be safely implanted in my brain. Because of my optimism, I wasn't frightened at all. I confidently placed my future in the hands of everyone in that room.

Sham Surgery

In spite of Lynda's optimism, she learned a year later that she had been in the control group and had not received a transplant. In order to rule out a placebo effect, the researchers sought to compare results of surgery with implants against fake or "sham" surgery. Lynda and nineteen other participants had holes drilled in their heads but did not receive cell transplants during the surgery.

For a few months, Lynda said she actually felt some improvement, but it was short lasting, and after about 4 months, she realized her symptoms were worsening. She was relieved to learn at the end of the year that she hadn't received the implant—this meant that her hope for improvement was still alive. As part of the research protocol she was given the opportunity to receive actual implant surgery, which took place about 2 years later, in 1998.

Promising Results: The Basis for More Research

Lynda wrote in July 1999:

Good news from New York!

Just want to let everyone know about the get-together at Columbia Presbyterian in New York City on Sunday afternoon, July 11th. It was for all the people who are participating in Drs. Freed and Fahn's fetal-transplant study. Finally, after being cautioned against talking with each other before the results were released, we were invited to get together to meet and hear the latest results.

Although the results in general seem to be better for those under age 60, they did speak of good results happening for the over-60 group, but at a slower rate. One 75-year-old man experienced very good results, they said.

Out of 19 who received the "right" surgery the first time, one person is off meds altogether and three are taking very small amounts now. The greatest improvements occur at the 12- to 18-month post-op time and continue from there.

PET scans show that all transplanted cells *did* grow in the recipient's brain. Why they work better in some than in others is a good question and will hopefully be the basis for one of the next studies.

Dr. Freed said he had hoped this surgery would be the answer to PD. Instead of feeling that his hopes for a medical miracle weren't realized, he knows that so much valuable information has been obtained and is already being used for future research.

I had the opportunity to see the doctors and nurses who have worked so hard to make this study work. They are dedicated, caring, and wonderful people who only want to see PD ended. I have the utmost respect for them and always will. I say "thank you" to them every time I get out of bed by myself, turn over in bed *all by myself*, and accomplish those little things taken for granted by so many.

Update: October 1999

Lynda McKenzie wrote on 26 October 1999:

It has been almost a year since the "real" surgery for me (December 1998). The majority of my days are "on" now, as opposed to this time last year when the majority were "off." Since February, I haven't had the incredible dystonia I once had.

The past 2 weeks have been a whirlwind for me; in fact, the past few months have just flown by! We have traveled to Vancouver, Nova Scotia, Maine, New York City, Montréal, and Ottawa. I have been interviewed on numerous TV stations here in Canada, as well as many radio shows.

I have resumed driving, and no longer have that awful feeling wondering if even if I get there, will I get home? Dyskinesia has decreased as well; my bruises are actually healing and not being replaced! I know that the positive results from the surgery weren't as quick as I'd hoped (we all have our dreams), but now, looking back on the past year, they are definitely here.

I feel as though I've been given a second chance. Each day is a new discovery, and I look forward to continuing to improve.

I know that the surgery I had is not the cure, or even the perfect solution for everyone, but it is an important step on the way. I want to be part of the solution, and not being a doctor or a scientist or a researcher, I feel that I can do my part by giving PD some visibility. I really want to keep hope alive, and I believe that by getting out there and speaking, and increasing awareness, I can do that.

A Letter from Lynda: August 2000

Al and I just returned from my 18-month post-op tests in New York City. The news is not particularly earth-shattering on that front. As the results continue to be tallied from the remaining participants, it is becoming more and more obvious that the fetal tissue implant surgery is just a step in the right direction, not an end in itself.

Granted, some people are feeling better, and that is wonderful. I wish I were one of those who are sure they improved measurably. I do know that now the pressure is off and people aren't looking for me to show up one day completely cured.... My physical symptoms are as manageable as 13-year-old Parkinson's can be, but the remarkable thing is my emotional well-being. And that is just as good, if not better than ever. There is no need for me to second guess every tremor, every episode of dyskinesia or rigidity, as to why? How? Or when? They just are. That also doesn't mean I never get frustrated, or upset, or cry. I do. But that's all right, because it's part of the package. A package I can accept and deal with. It isn't what I'd wish for in a perfect world, but it's okay and it's me.

As Al and I retrieved our car from the hospital parking lot and deposited our bags inside, we realized that it was exactly 4 years ago, almost to the day, that we were there for my very first series of tests after being accepted into the study. How excited and full of promise we both felt then! I was positive that this procedure would provide the "out" for me from the clutches of this disease. I also was so sure I would receive the right tissue the first time. I kept picturing myself whizzing through the tests, astounding everyone with my vast improvement and ultimately becoming a spokesperson for the procedure.

However, so far, I have to admit that some things, no matter how badly you want them, are just not meant to be....

In March 2001, the results of this pioneering study were published in the *New England Journal of Medicine*. The researchers found evidence that transplanted embryonic neurons survived in the brains of a majority of the subjects of all ages; however, measurable clinical benefits were realized only by patients under 60 years old. The researchers concluded that surgical techniques needed further refinement, due to the occurrence of serious dystonia and dyskinesia in five patients receiving the transplants.[6]

Dr. Freed indicated that the research "...will continue, for we now have a base of experience.... This research is an important milepost for the ongoing development of cell transplantation as a treatment for Parkinson's. We are now testing ways to produce a better and more uniform response in individual patients."[7]

Although there were some negative reports in the mass media, calling the fetal tissue transplant study a "failure," Lynda McKenzie did not share that viewpoint. She stated, "When people look at me now and hear that I was part of Dr Freed's study, I can see them shake their heads as they think 'Hmm, so that was obviously a waste of time' and 'those poor patients who were given those promises and false hopes.' Wrong, wrong, wrong! First of all, who knows what we would be like now had we not been part of the study. Secondly, look how much we learned to enable us to go on to subsequent studies."[8]

Lynda also indicated if given the opportunity, she would have the transplant treatment all over again, and she looks forward to the future and the promise of a cure for Parkinson's.

LYNDA The past 4 years have been the most incredible 4 years of my life! So much has happened! So many doors have opened, I've met so many wonderful people, so many roadblocks have turned into opportunities—how could I even dare to wish it hadn't happened? If I were given a chance to relive these past 4 years, would I have chosen any differently? Nope. I'd do it again in a minute.

This summer finds me busy with many things. I'm exploring several alternative methods of dealing with Parkinson's, including a type of Reiki, massage, regular exercise, meditation, neurofeedback, nutrition, visiting special friends, and just chillin' out. Maybe that's why I'm feeling pretty good.

Even though part of my brain has suffered from corporate downsizing in the dopamine department, I'm convinced that there is some other course (or courses) of action excitedly waiting in the wings. Because I'm the way I am, I'd like to be there when it makes its debut.

Given the choice of being a realist who slams the door shut, lamenting that something "probably won't work," or an optimist who opens the door with a wide welcome and sees how it *could* work, I know what I'll continue to pick.

chapter 8

Routes to a Cure, Hopes for the Future

A Voice in the Park...A Piece of Cloth

DAVID BOOTS

I live in a small "granny unit" across a small creek from a public park. During the wet winter months, there's very little activity. As warmer weather approaches, the sound of horseshoes, the laughter of children, and the crack of baseball bats begin to be part of my daily symphony. (I almost expect sometimes to see my Mom drive up in a Chevrolet to hand me an apple pie.)

In the evening when there's a baseball game, the bright lights by the field and the muffled voices of the loudspeakers filter through the trees to my place, where I'm (most likely) lying down. I sometimes like to think of this as "the voice of God," words spoken with volume and authority that I can't decipher.

At times, I like to believe that this voice is telling me that things will be alright and not to give up believing in myself...that I already know what I can give of myself each day...that my actions (or lack thereof) as a "PD-surfer" are both an experience for me to learn from, as well as an opportunity to make others aware and educate the masses. When my meds kick in, this voice loses its magical quality and sounds again like a night game at the park.

I'm not religious but I found myself in an odd predicament: unable to let go (literally) of something a friend gave me. I met this person at the last bluegrass festival I performed (banjo) at before the band "let me go" due to the PD and its effect on my playing. I'd shared some banjo knowledge with this young teenager at the festival and we traded addresses to stay in contact. My PD was never brought up till months later when he asked me in a letter to tape some of my "live playing" for him. It has often been difficult for me to tell others about the PD. I didn't know what to do other than tell this 15-year-old my situation and hope that he understood.

I didn't get another letter from him for almost three months; I didn't expect to. When his letter arrived, there was a brief note inside and a piece of black-and-white checkered cloth in a small folded square. The front of his note told me about a banjo contest he'd recently placed second in and that he was looking forward to driving a car soon, but the back had this on it: "David, My Mom and I prayed a long time over this piece of cloth. It says in the Bible that if you pray over a piece of cloth and give it to a person who is ill, they will be cured of their sickness." I held that piece of cloth the rest of the afternoon. I still have it in my wallet and can't bring myself to stop carrying it. I was taken aback by my friend's "gift" to me and touched by his words. My pallidotomy is scheduled for sometime next month, and I'm sure that piece of cloth will be there with me.[1]

Hopes and Dreams for "The Cure"

If we all do everything we can to eradicate this disease, in my 50s I'll be dancing at my children's weddings. And mine will be just one of millions of happy stories.
MICHAEL J. FOX[2]

Diagnosed with Parkinson's last year at age 47, I have a dream. I see myself at 60 with the disease process reversed/cured. I'll still be an educator, and, I hope, enjoying my grandchildren, and watching the latest hit by a lively Michael J. Fox. JEANETTE FUHR

JERRY FINCH, TEXAS I'm not going to be the only one who looks to tomorrow with more than a spark of hope. "A couple of years down the road," they said. "A cure for Parkinson's," they added. So close, yet so very far away.

And I'm not the only one who will say a prayer of thanks for those scientists and researchers who have devoted so much time and effort on our behalf. We aren't there yet, but with our combined effort, there will be a time when we can shrug off this cloak of Parkinson's and get on with our lives. "A cure..." Is it really possible?

DENNIS GREENE, AUSTRALIA The grand strategies that will win this war are beyond us as individuals. New drugs, new surgical techniques, and new genetic information—these are the things that will win the war against Parkinson's disease. We individual foot soldiers can only approach the war piecemeal, one skirmish, one day, at a time. It is our task to secure our own piece of the battleground.

DON BERNS, PENNSYLVANIA We are joined in the battle with PD to "ease the burden and to find a cure" by the likes of Billy Graham, the pope, Janet Reno, and the former heavyweight champion of the world, who know that PD represents only a temporary defeat. Together with neuroscientists, doctors, politicians, and the people affected by PD, we stand poised to defeat this foe as we enter the new millennium.

A Cure: Why Now?

DENNIS GREENE I too would like to see a cure in my lifetime, but I have never quite worked out why so may of us seem to think it *must* happen in time to save *this* generation—what's so special about us?

...Because by One Stroke of the Pen

BERNARD SHAW, AUSTRIA I am a positive-thinking person, and I have much patience, but when I think of how long it has been since James Parkinson placed all the known facts in front of the world—yet there's still no cure; the mind boggles. In the last 100 years, we have had two world wars and many smaller wars. When I think of what these wars alone have cost, I see red; when I think of the paltry research funding for cures (not just for Parkinson's), my blood begins to boil. But who am I to think that some of my words might reach any of the people in power, that by one stroke of the pen we could fund research so that a cure could be found?

...Because We're Bearing the Fruits of Earlier Research

BOB MARTONE, TEXAS In 1982, somewhere in Santa Clara, California, several people began showing up at local hospitals with uncontrollable movements, paralysis, and a variety of other symptoms resembling Parkinson's disease. An alert young doctor of neurology, Bill Langston, recognizing the symptoms, and with the help of the local police and the FBI, was able to trace the cause of this terribly incapacitating illness to a drug that had been manufactured by a chemist in his garage, then sold as synthetic heroin for considerable profit.

Those people's misfortunes and that chemist's miscalculation have been the catalyst for much of the successful research performed on Parkinson's disease over the last 10 years. That drug, called MPTP, destroys certain brain cells that are also destroyed by Parkinson's disease. The chemist's terrible mistake has enabled scientists to re-create Parkinson's symptoms in laboratory animals. The scientists are now able to perform research that before was not possible on human beings. As a result, a cure for Parkinson's disease may be found much sooner.

...Because There's Real Hope

BARBARA MALLUT, CALIFORNIA In the 3 years since my surgery [1994–1997], the world of medical research has *finally* started bringing out new drugs to ease Parkinson's symptoms. In these 3 short years (*long* years if you're awaiting a cure!), I've read about dynamic exploration and mapping of the brain, and this offers me hope that in the relatively near future this beast of a disease will be tamed.

...Because the Cure for PD Will Lead to Other Cures

Gerald D. Fischbach, M.D., director of the National Institute of Neurological Disorders and Stroke, stated at a Senate Appropriations Committee hearing, "Beyond the impact on Parkinson's disease itself, Parkinson's research will certainly lead to insights about many other diseases in which nerve cells die.... Most notable are the classic chronic neurodegenerative diseases such as Alzheimer's, Huntington's, and ALS [amyotrophic lateral sclerosis, or Lou Gehrig's disease]. Many devastating neurodegenerative disorders also attack the brain of infants and children. Nerve cell death is critical in stroke, brain and spinal cord injury, and in epilepsy.[3]

...Because We Can Stop the Suffering and Reduce the Economic Cost

PHIL TOMPKINS, NEW JERSEY/MASSACHUSETTS Regarding the urgency, I understand two aspects. First, there is the personal. I do not want to suffer in my old age, nor do I want anyone else to, if it can be avoided.

Second is a cost-benefit projection. The figures that have been developed show that the costs of developing and administering the "cure" therapies will be significantly less than the costs of *having* PD under the present modes of therapy.

...Because Annually, Parkinson's Disease Costs the U.S. Economy:

▶ $25,000 per year for every PWP (total annual societal and family costs, based on 1994 dollars);

▶ $39,000 per year for every PWP under the age of 65 (yearly earnings loss due to PD);[4]

A total of $25 billion per year.

How Do We Define "The Cure"?

What exactly is meant by "finding the cure"? Can a person be "healed" without being cured of the disease? Should we look beyond traditional medical science for the answers to these questions?

DENNIS GREENE One of the things that strikes me about The Cure is how often it is mentioned, yet how seldom, if ever, it is defined. Just what constitutes a cure for PD? For that matter, just what constitutes a cure? My dictionary defines "cure" as:

1. to get rid of an ailment;
2. to restore to health.

At first glance, this seems straightforward enough—but is it? By either of those definitions, we do not have a cure for PD if, however well controlled the symptoms are, they will come crashing back the moment we stop treatment. PD is only cured if after an action or sequence of actions the disease and its symptoms are eradicated without need for further intervention.

This removes the newer DBS-type surgical interventions from the list of possible cures. However refined they get—however good the results—they will no more cure PD than an artificial leg cures the amputation of a real leg. At best, they may come to be a very good substitute for a cure—for those who can afford them, and who live in countries with the technology and expertise to perform them.

So it seems to me that before we can say we are cured, we need to have found a way to restore natural dopamine production in the brain. To achieve this, a way must be found to successfully replace the missing cells of the substantia nigra or of successfully regrowing them. The only other cure I can see is finding what causes PD and stopping it before it starts.

SANDRA NORRIS, NORTH CAROLINA   A cure is nice to think about, to dream about. Knowing I have lived this day to the fullest of my capabilities—have accomplished some, if not all, that I set out to do—brings me closer to a cure. The "cure" to me is knowing that the PD has not beat me today and that I may lay my head down tonight knowing that although the war still rages, I won the round for today.

BARBARA BLAKE-KREBS, KANSAS   Upon hearing the diagnosis of PD and learning the implications of that diagnosis, something within us besides the physical dopamine-producing cells is attacked. Often our very innermost concept of self and self-worth is impaired and needs to be healed. Ridding our air of toxins—chemical (body) and psychological (mind)—appears to me to make sense, and may need to be accomplished at both the personal and societal levels.

BARBARA RAGER, ONTARIO, CANADA   Since I've been on this journey, I've started to turn all my attention to the process of healing. I've found that I personally can contribute significantly to this process. I read inspirational books. I keep friends close to me who are positive, optimistic, and willing to share both their own as well as my suffering, without giving advice.

I have looked into alternative healing practices—the effects of vitamins, nutrition, and homeopathic remedies. I am developing an excellent rapport with my neuro, whom I respect and trust. I try to find objectivity by writing about my contact with the world through this disease. I take time to learn about PD from a medical point of view so I can try to visualize the healing. And I've reworked my priority list to include actively loving myself at the top. This space is a little small in my daily life, as I have not given it much consideration in the past.

BARBARA BLAKE-KREBS One February evening, in 2001, I received three successive phone calls to turn on the CBS-affiliate local news, which had announced an upcoming feature on PD. It was a report of a collaborative research project between the University of Kansas Medical Center (KUMC) and Dr. Michael Greene, chiropractor and acupuncturist, on the effects of an acupuncture program he is using.

The 6-month study was initiated in response to patient interest in this alternative treatment for Parkinson's symptoms. According to Greene, during a routine checkup, Dr. Raj Pahwa, director of the Parkinson Disease and Movement Disorder Center, noted marked improvement in a patient receiving acupuncture treatments. One participant said he expected it might take up to 2 years for benefits to become evident. Greene is enthusiastically training other area acupuncturists in the nuances of this program, and patients have formed a special support group.

In speaking to Dr. Greene the next day, I learned that he had a dream too—through a course of acupuncture treatments to help enable each patient's body to heal itself.

DENNIS GREENE My belief and experience is that the miracle of healing *does* occur, but it doesn't involve setting aside the laws of the universe. It occurs where all miracles occur, in our hearts and minds, and it enables us to say, only half in jest, "There is nothing wrong with me that a cure for Parkinson's won't fix."

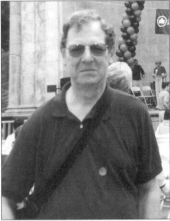

Phil Tompkins at the 2000 New York
City Unity Walk

LINDA HERMAN

Remaining Hopeful

PHIL TOMPKINS Despite the
fact that the age of onset is
decreasing, despite the fact that
PD remains poorly understood
by the public at large, and
despite the fact that my PD and
your PD don't go away but just
get worse as time passes, I
remain hopeful that ways to
arrest and reverse PD are immi-
nent. I remain hopeful because
of recent trends like these:

▶ The brain-research effort as a
whole, and research in neuro-
degenerative diseases in particular, has increased, partly due to
the "Decade of the Brain" program, partly because that's where
a lot of the excitement in medical research is these days.

▶ Research efforts in diseases associated with aging have
increased, largely due to the increasing proportion of older
people in the population.

▶ Considerable progress in PD research has been made in a
relatively short time.

▶ New companies that produce medicines based on research in
such areas as neurotrophic growth factors and genetic engineering have sprung up, and these medicines are now under-
going clinical trials.

We shouldn't just sit back and wait for the results of all the above
—we still need to work for more funding, better public understanding, etc. I just want to give some reasons for hanging in there.

Routes to a Cure

At the beginning of the twenty-first century, the most promising routes to a cure for PD include the following:

1. Understanding the interaction of genetic and environmental factors that may trigger the onset of Parkinson's.

2. Developing new biological agents that protect healthy nerve cells and others that will restore function to already stricken cells.

3. Replacing nonfunctioning nerve cells with healthy cells and developing a viable source for these cells.

Environmental Factors

Exposure to agricultural pesticides, as well as commonly used household and garden insecticides, hydrocarbon solvents (found in petroleum-based paints and glues), heavy metals, and well water are all currently under investigation as risk factors for PD. The resulting biochemical changes in dopamine-producing cells exposed to pesticides are also under investigation in the laboratory. Identifying and better understanding the mechanism of neural cell damage will open new pathways to the prevention, detection, and treatment of many neurological conditions.

Vietnam War and Persian Gulf War veterans exposed to very high levels of neurotoxins have been reported to have a higher rate of Parkinson's and other neurological conditions than the general population.

In the September 2000 issue of the *Archives of Neurology*, University of Texas researchers reported that brain scans of some veterans suffering from Gulf War Syndrome did show evidence of cell damage. Additionally, blood tests for dopamine activity indicated that these vets had higher levels of dopamine production. The researchers hypothesized that "the remaining cells have to work extra hard to produce dopamine and may burn out and die prematurely, resulting in the movement problems seen in some of the vets...and that the vets who display the brain damage and dopamine abnormality may be at risk down the road for developing Parkinson's disease or similar conditions."[5]

Related studies are currently being funded by the U.S. Department of Defense's Neurotoxin Exposure Research Treatment Program. Insights into the role of toxins in brain-cell degeneration and dopamine production gained from this research may help unravel the puzzle of Parkinson's disease and lead to improved treatments.

RUDY WEST, VIRGINIA I do not believe we can point to a single event or factor as being the specific cause, but in seeking probable or suspected causes—in my own case and that of other Vietnam veterans—the evidence is strong that neurotoxins (chemical herbicides, pesticides, insecticides, repellants, in addition to Agent Orange) were a contributing factor. There are similar subtle (but real) symptoms showing up in Gulf War veterans. Anyone who is familiar with the exposure symptoms to neurotoxins can see them very plainly.

CHARLIE MEYER, WISCONSIN In addition to toxins such as pesticides, there are a whole group of other environmental factors—infections, in utero factors, diet, exercise, climate, emotional stressors, medications, sun exposure, sleep, etc. I do think toxins are a good bet, but they are only one of many possibilities. I really hope research comes up with something irrefutable. We owe that to our children.

JOHN BJORK, WEST VIRGINIA

:-) Dateline: "Parkinsaw," Michigan :-)

There has been much discussion everywhere about the causes of Parkinson's. We have reported before that as far as we can figure out up this way, it could just as well be the subpar play of the Detroit Tigers causing excessive pressure on dopamine-producing cells as anything else. Still, there is also the potentially adverse impact on our brain cells from excessive exposure to the little temptations of life that could play a role in the matter.

For example, what about continual consumption of Twinkies as a child, with all that sugar, washed down by soda pop and Kool-Aid? How about sniffing glue in paper bags, which allowed you to fly your model plane after you built it? And how about rock and roll? Blame it on the Stones!

To tell the truth, I put my money on the environmental neurotoxin theory, especially involving pesticides and copper and iron in the water supply. (Especially since the Upper Peninsula was once a major producer of iron and copper ore.) That way, I don't have to worry about listening to Mick Jagger while I gobble down a couple of chocolate donuts. I've also heard it could be from faulty jeans; what, my Levi's were too ragged and frayed while I was growing up?

The Role of Genetics

Fueled by new discoveries in the field of molecular biology, such as the insights provided by the Human Genome Project, knowledge about the role of genetics in PD is rapidly advancing. Genetic researchers may soon be able to answer the question of why, under identical environmental conditions, some people develop PD while others escape unharmed.

In the 26 June 1997, issue of *Science* magazine, researchers reported the identification of an abnormal gene found in families with high occurrences of Parkinson's disease. Dr. Mihael Polymeropoulos and his colleagues at the National Human Genome Research Institute discovered a mutation in the gene coding for a protein found in brain cells called alpha-synuclein.

While only a small percentage of families are known to carry this gene, Dr. William Langston of the Parkinson's Institute predicted in 1999 that "its discovery will provide invaluable new clues on the causes of typical Parkinson's disease, and may lead to the identification of new proteins that are responsible for cell death."[6]

Indeed, the following year, Japanese scientists identified a mutation in a second gene, which they named "*parkin.*" They believed it might be associated with forms of early-onset PD. Researchers at Duke University later identified a second type of mutation in the *parkin* gene, which may aid in protein destruction but is found in people with later-onset PD. Discoveries such as these indicate the likelihood that PD is caused by an interaction of both genetic and environmental causes. An individual's genetic makeup may determine his or her susceptibility to neurological damage caused by various toxins.

Research continues on the roles of genetics and the environment in Parkinson's disease. Most researchers agree that understanding the causes of the disease will help hasten the discovery of a cure and help identify preventative measures. As Charlie Meyer wrote, "We owe that to our children."

JERRY FINCH   A side effect of this work might be that the discovery of these genes would lead to identification of those children who will, in a few years, develop PD. This identification would lead to starting whatever needs to be done so they never have to experience the Wonderful World of PD.

Knowing that a passed-on gene would cause my grandson to have PD when he turns 50 is something I don't even want to think about.... Now, through this research, there is a glimmer of hope that my grandson may never have to worry about what Grandpa passed along.

Now, if I could just get a couple thousand dollars of that money to explore my premise that the cure for PD involves BBQ....

Protecting and Restoring Nerve Cells

Another route to a cure involves developing new biological agents that protect healthy nerve cells (neuroprotective agents) and others that will restore function to already stricken cells (neurotrophic agents).

Oxidative damage to brain cells, similar to rust damage to metal, is believed to be the primary event leading to the onset and progression of Parkinson's and other neurodegenerative diseases. Alpha-synuclein proteins in brain cells (see the preceding section) have been identified as one of the targets of the oxidative stress. Researchers are investigating new antioxidant drugs and neuroprotective agents in an attempt to halt the oxidative damage. Being able to target a specific protein may pave the road to therapies that slow or reverse the progression of PD.

Restoring Damaged Neurons

As discussed in chapter 1, the symptoms of Parkinson's disease result from the degeneration and death of dopamine-producing cells in the substantia nigra area of the brain. Dopamine is a neurochemical transmitter, essential for smooth and normal movements. Symptoms become evident when the supply of dopamine is depleted about 80 percent below necessary levels. Several possible methods of restoring damaged neurons are currently under exploration:

1. Growth Factors: Turning Brain Cells Back On

DR. WILLIAM LANGSTON SAYS: A little-known fact I find with my patients is that while you have an 80 percent dopamine depletion—that means 80 percent of the dopamine is gone, or more, by the time you get Parkinson's—*only about 60 percent of the cells are gone.* What does that mean?

It means that there are a lot of cells still there that aren't doing their job; they're not pulling their weight. Growth factors, conceivably, could turn those cells back on. And that's where the excitement is. That could be surgery without the surgery.[7]

Immunophilin Ligands

Immunophilin ligands, tiny proteins small enough to pass through the blood-brain barrier, are under study as a potential orally administered growth factor that could stimulate brain-cell growth.

A human clinical trial is currently underway to evaluate the safety and efficacy of this treatment. Researchers have expressed hope that it could prove to be the first medicine to regenerate damaged nerve cells in the brain, and could eventually be used to treat PD as well as other brain disorders.

2. Gene Therapy

In the fall of 2000, Dr. Jeffrey Kordower of Rush Presbyterian Medical Center reported success with another form of restorative therapy. Using a virus as the transport, genes for dopamine production were transferred into the brains of monkeys with MPTP-induced Parkinson's symptoms (see page 189). These genes prompted brain cells to produce more dopamine, and three of the five treated monkeys were totally relieved of Parkinson's symptoms.[8] Further animal testing is currently underway, and human clinical trials might begin in 3 to 5 years. Gene therapy may become another hopeful route to a cure.

Stem-Cell Transplantation

In February 2001, Dr. Ole Isacson of Harvard Medical School and Dr. Ronald McKay of the NIH announced that by grafting embryonic rodent stem cells into the brains of mice and rats with induced Parkinson's symptoms, they were able to restore normal movements and functioning.[9]

Stem cells are like building blocks. At the earliest stages of development, they have the potential to become virtually any type of tissue. These cells can be isolated and manipulated in the lab to develop into specialized cells, such as muscle cells, blood cells—or dopamine-producing brain cells. An NIH fact sheet states that stem-cell research "promises new treatments and possibly even cures for many debilitating diseases and injuries, including Parkinson's disease, diabetes, heart disease, multiple sclerosis, burns and spinal cord injuries."[10]

The cells currently used in this research are derived from unused embryos from fertility treatments and would otherwise die, be destroyed, or be frozen indefinitely. Additional sources of viable stem cells are under investigation.

Researchers predict that human trials of stem-cell therapy could begin this year; however, U.S. federal research funding is threatened by intense controversies over the use of human embryonic stem cells. Many PWPs believe that stem-cell research could lead to a cure in the not-so-distant future and fear that their hopes for a Parkinson's-free life could be smashed by political and religious pressure groups. The research is expected to continue, however, in other countries.

PHIL TOMPKINS The National Institutes of Health have published guidelines which ensure that the embryos from which stem cells are extracted with government funding are created for no other purpose than to treat infertility. The guidelines also prevent creating embryos for profit or for use by designated recipients. Donation requires the informed consent of the donors. Extraction of stem cells is not the violation of human life that the critics contend it to be. The embryos from which the cells are extracted are developmentally less than one week old. They have not been and will not be implanted into a woman's uterus. They are not on the way to becoming an infant.

There are politicians and clergymen who oppose stem-cell research and treatment. What a crime it would be to sacrifice the health of millions of Americans to the views of a vocal minority.

JEANETTE FUHR, MISSOURI I would like any person who opposes stem-cell research to consider the possibility that, cured of Parkinson's, juvenile diabetes, Alzheimer's, or Lou Gehrig's, there are human beings who can have a better, more productive life. Scrapping excess embryos from in vitro fertilization is as wasteful and inhumane as not donating organs of deceased individuals to save and improve the lives of human recipients.

MARYHELEN DAVILA, ARIZONA I am a long-term young-onset PD (diagnosed 13 years ago). I was a member of the list for a long while, and did what I could against PD. My PD's progression has been nasty, taking more and more from me, including my ability to communicate by e-mail (this note took hours). It forced me to draw back—go off the list, refrain from support groups, end my volunteer and fund-raising activities. It's been one-on-one. No winner yet…but the party's not over yet, and I still want to dance. My contributions might fall short, but I'm not throwing in the towel. I believe in miracles. I want to encourage stem-cell research.

The Knockout Blow to PD

KEES PAAP, THE NETHERLANDS/TEXAS I am searching for the best possible way to cope for the next 5 years, because I am convinced that I will be one of the lucky people who will be cured of this awful illness. Until that time, I try to have the best quality of life as is reasonable to expect. I want to be cured, and I want to live as a normal citizen in the United States, to work the 15 years I lost to PD.

PHIL GESOTTI, VIRGINIA I have a lot of people depending on me. My loving wife deserves to have companionship—not a burden—during retirement years. My children deserve my time for teaching, travel, play, and, most importantly, love. My community deserves a place where their children can safely have fun and enjoy the rewards of hard work. My company deserves the benefit of my years of experience and problem-solving skills. I'm not giving up. I will fight to the end!

DON BERNS Taking our cue from the Champ, who showed us how "to float like a butterfly and sting like a bee," we are ready to remove the sting from the bee of PD so that we can fly like butterflies.

Bringing together our resources, we will continue our search for the cure whether it be found through transplants, implants, neural growth factors, gene therapy, or new medicines. We will deliver the knockout blow to Parkinson's disease.

Hopes from the Creative Team of *When Parkinson's Strikes Early*

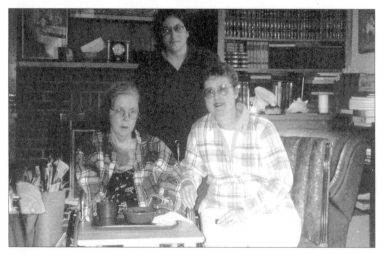

Barbara Blake-Krebs, Jeanette Fuhr, and Linda Herman (standing) meet in-person for the first time (November 2000)

The Importance of "Nobodies" Having a Dream

Barbara Blake-Krebs

Thank you, kind reader, for looking at these pages. It may surprise you that a cure for and the prevention of Parkinson's is not my fondest dream. That would be something even more complicated and universal: love and joy in every earthling's heart and the ability to work together and live peaceably.

I don't recall truly having a dream—a goal—as a young person. Maybe I was just too self-satisfied. I was blessed with a loving middle-class family in America and a good education.

The year 1977 marks one turning point in my life. At age 36, I entered graduate school in the field of broadcasting. I give serendipity credit for what happened next. In February I spotted a notice of a meeting for anyone interested in having alternative community radio in the greater Kansas City area. Eleven years later, at 10 A.M. on Sunday, 28 February 1988, as board president and general manager, I welcomed listeners to the first broadcast day of a new hundred-thousand-watt FM community station. KKFI came to be by a handful of wonderful people—nobodies—with a dream and a lot of determination.

In 1985, my mom was cured of breast cancer, while I added Parkinson's disease to my identity. In the 1990s, my mobility and independence started to wane. Then one day in 1995, my professorial husband brought home what I at first viewed as an expensive new toy—a brand new Mac with Internet access. I soon fell in love with my Mac!

Soon after, I joined PIEN, heard about the dream for a cure, and became an advocate. The past two years of compiling the stories of our fellow PWPs and of documenting the rise of patient advocates—nobodies—has been one of the richest times of my life. Lessons learned go far beyond setting the stage for curing a pathological disease or diseases.

This has been truly a model for learning through the Internet about the hidden lives behind the masks of all of us who belong to the family of humankind; the symptoms and diagnoses of societies' breakdown(s); understanding the components and possible progression(s); identifying temporary solutions and possible routes to a cure. As is the case for many PWPs, invisibility and isolation keep us apart and in the dark. Jim Cordy put his finger on the best part of the patient-advocate experience: "I thought once I would never have friendships as strong as those I formed in the cauldron of my college career. But I see it is the experience of being thrown together sharing the same vulnerability and purpose that is the main ingredient."

Three Hopes

Linda Herman

I was diagnosed on 4 December 1995. I think many of us will always remember the exact date and circumstances and the exact words spoken by our doctors on that day. I recall being told about all the research going on, and that there was good reason to be optimistic. I try to be.

My first hope for the future is that our children will never hear the life-altering words "You have Parkinson's disease"—not at any age.

My second hope is that when "the cure" is found, it will be available to every PWP who could benefit from it—not only those who can pay for it. For those who cannot be cured, I hope more effective treatments will improve the quality of their lives.

My third hope is that in the future, no one will be forced to relinquish their dreams to Parkinson's or any other chronic disease—whether that dream is to educate the young, run a family business, compete in sports, make music, star in a TV show, or be elected to their nation's highest office.

The Blessing of Hope

Jeanette Fuhr *(Our day-to-day cheerleader and the godmother to this book)*

As I sit at my computer this morning, I am amazed at the blessings in my life. After weeks of dry weather, the sky has opened and rain is coming down and restoring the soil with moisture. I feel like the dry earth must feel when the rain washes down. I am showered with encouragement from my friends who, like me, struggle to find the silver lining to the cloud of Parkinson's disease.

This same month, 4 years ago, when I heard my neurologist tell me, "You may have Parkinson's disease, although at 47, you're too young," I felt like I had just been punched in the stomach. I'd never known anyone with Parkinson's disease, and as the doctor talked to me and my husband about the medication he was prescribing, the probable 15 to 20 good years most people with Parkinson's enjoy, the numerous new surgical interventions being tried, I only half heard his words. I was relieved that the MRI, blood tests, etc., ruled out stroke, a tumor, or other deadly diagnoses, but I still wondered, "Why do I have Parkinson's disease?"

Four years later, I still have no definite answer to that question. What I know about Parkinson's has grown tenfold. I have met people with Parkinson's. People my parents' age or in their 50s have been at the support group I attend. People my own age have been "introduced" via the PIEN (Parkinson's Information Exchange Network), and I have "met" more young-onset PWPs through reading their stories in national magazines, especially since the *People* magazine article interviewing Michael J. Fox, who is even younger than I and who has had the disease since age 30. All of us have things in common.

We have been diagnosed with a chronic, incurable brain disease. We are not sure how this disease will affect us, our families, our communities. But one thing each of us must have in order to keep getting up and facing each day is the support of others and the hope that the future holds promise of finding the cause of and the treatment/prevention/cure for Parkinson's.

When I sit down with family this Thanksgiving, I am thankful for the blessings that shower down on me like the rain falls on the parched ground. I want to soak up the blessings of love, health, prosperity, well-being, and that all-important blessing of *hope*. For without hope, my life and yours would not be worth anything.

TO OUR READERS: *By purchasing this book, you have already helped to find the cure for Parkinson's disease. All royalties will be donated to Parkinson's research and to programs that provide care and improve the lives of Parkinson's patients. The authors and the more than 2,000 members of the Parkinson's Information Exchange Network (PIEN) thank you for your support.*

About Our Contributors

The following contributors to When Parkinson's Strikes Early *would like to add a few more words about themselves and living with Parkinson's.*

BARBARA BLAKE-KREBS has a Master's Degree in Communication from the University of Missouri. Her professional life includes working as an international educational program specialist, writing and researching community studies, public relations, and teaching. Besides being the originator/producer of an ongoing weekly public affairs show in 1989 on KKFI 90.1 FM, she also spent 11 years helping to develop the full-powered community radio station for the greater Kansas City area and was general manager for 3 years. Diagnosed with Parkinson's disease in 1984, Barbara has worked since 1996 with others to develop public awareness and support for a cure. Since 1996, she has written a column, "Wit and Wisdom on the Internet," for the local Parkinson's newsletter in Kansas City. She lives with her husband in Merriam, Kansas.

LINDA HERMAN has a Master's of Library Science degree from the State University of New York at Buffalo, and has worked as an academic librarian for the past 17 years. She is currently Technical Services Librarian at Medaille College in Buffalo, New York. Linda is also a freelance researcher and has been a community advocate for inclusive education for students with disabilities. Her life changed irrevocably at age 45 when she was diagnosed with Parkinson's disease, commonly considered a disease of the elderly. It changed again when she discovered the Parkinson's Information Exchange Network, where she met "Parkie" advocates from around the globe. Linda resides in Amherst, New York, with her husband, who is also an academic librarian. They have two children who are currently attending college and graduate school.

KEN AIDEKMAN is vice president of an asset management firm and lives in Short Hills, New Jersey, with his wife, Ellen, and children, Matthew and Andrea. Ken's interest in curing Parkinson's stems from having both a grandfather and father who were diagnosed with the disease. He assisted Margot Zobel with the formation of the Parkinson's Unity Walk in New York City and was the organization's first Chairman. Ken currently serves on the Board of Directors of the Parkinson Alliance.

RICK L. BARRETT, 39, is a civil engineer specializing in forensics and expert witness testimony. As a structures specialist, he took part in the rescue efforts following the 1995 bombing of the Oklahoma City federal building. Rick retired last year and spends his time raising his two young children, Nolan and Holly. He writes, "It has taken me a long while to find peace with my condition, especially losing my expectations of the future. Now I live each day more fully with the support of those around me and hope that the future will bring a cure." Rick looks forward to sharing his life with his new bride, Victoria, and her son, Clinton.

JEANA BARTLETT, PD onset at age 33, is a mother and home-maker in Georgia. At 48, she has had both a pallidotomy and deep brain stimulation. Originally from an agricultural area in Southeast Missouri, she feels that toxic exposure to pesticides may have caused her Parkinson's. Jeana writes, "I could not have made it through these years alone. My doctors, husband, sons, family, friends, and my faith have been my mainstay."

EMMA BENNION, from Norfolk, United Kingdom, has served as Chairperson of YAPP&Rs, the young-onset special interest group of the Parkinson's Disease Society, and on the PDS Board of Trustees. She writes, "I am particularly interested in education and communication and enjoy talking to all PWPs, especially the young who are newly diagnosed and frightened. I hope that my positive attitude has, in some small way, helped others to come to terms with this dreadful condition."

JOHN BJORK was diagnosed 20 years ago at age 42. He retired from the U.S. Secret Service in 1994, following a 32-year career, and now resides in West Virginia. John is the creator of *The*

Parkinsaw Chronicle—humorous stories about "Parkinsaw," an imaginary community in Michigan's Upper Peninsula composed mostly of PWPs. See his website: www.mikeauldridge-.com/parknsaw.htm

DAVID BOOTS, from Northern California, is a self-proclaimed "rebel without a pause." His stories (many of which are found on his web page (<http://www.sonic.net/~bootst3k>) capture the many facets of PD and show his determination in trying not to let the disease get the best of him (or his characters).

PERRY D. COHEN, PH.D., is a health care consultant in Washington, D.C. He and his wife, Rosalie, are parents to college students, Shayna and Jonah. Diagnosed in 1996, Perry writes, "My first 50 years were training for my most important role—to work with PD advocates to end PD as we know it." His work currently focuses on moving clinical research from science to cures that reach PWP and fostering coordination among PD organizations.

MARYHELEN DAVILA, 48, lives in Phoenix, Arizona. At age 37, she was diagnosed with PD, but only after having seen four neurologists. She traces symptoms back to age 22. "I understood what I have to do, what we must do," she says. "It is as though each of us has a brick. Each brick has its place in the wall. Together we can build the wall that will stop PD and keep it back."

BOB DOLEZAL is from Tucson, father of two, and currently serves as Arizona APDA president. Diagnosed 9 years ago at age 56, he says, "I am not proud to have Parkinson's, but I am proud of how I live with it." As a Parkinson's advocate, he convinced an influential senator to take a lead role in supporting increased PD research funding. Bob adds, "Reading my 'Ode to Ali' at a hospital dedication in 1998, hugging Ali, was a lifetime experience."

JERRY FINCH was diagnosed with Parkinson's in 1990. "It's probably the best thing that happened to me. I was finally able to step off the fast track and start enjoying life, doing those things that I feel are truly important." Jerry operates a nonprofit organization, Habitat for Horses, that uses rescued horses to bring abused children back to life. His goal is to build a sanctuary of safety for horses and families suffering from abuse.

JEANETTE FUHR is a part-time instructor at a community college in Missouri. She is hopeful that awareness and funding for PD research will advance due to the shared experiences of hers and others with the disease. She also thanks her husband, Leo, and their two children, Brian and Brenda, for their support.

PHIL GESOTTI is a 51-year-old electrical engineer from Northern Virginia. He was diagnosed at age 46 and continues to work full time. Phil writes, "I am happily married to a wonderful loving woman who has been the sunshine of my life for over 18 years. We have the blessing of two teenage daughters who keep us young. I am working on a device that may potentially alleviate symptoms. Not bad for an old boy from West Virginia, eh?"

JOY GRAHAM cares for her husband, Bob, who was diagnosed with PD in 1990 on his 50th birthday. They served for 10 years on the committee of the Parkinson's Association of Western Australia. Joy edited the group's newsletter and created a video, *Lost Voices*, about the management of late-stage PD. They are now "retired" and enjoy living near the ocean in Fremantle, Australia.

DENNIS GREENE was diagnosed 14 years ago, at age 37. He was born in England, raised in Rhodesia (now Zimbabwe), and currently lives with his family in Perth, Australia. Dennis worked as a meteorologist, debt collector, soldier, and retail manager until PD forced him to retire. He is now very active in the PD community and recently coedited *Voices from the Parking Lot*, a compilation of writings about PD.

JO GREENE, Dennis's wife, is originally from Guernsey in the Channel Islands. She is a registered nurse, currently working with dementia sufferers. Jo and Dennis have two children.

LINDA GREULICH, from Ontario, California, was diagnosed at age 45 in 1994. She was the advertising manager for a large paper, with goals of becoming a publisher, but is now on permanent disability. Linda writes, "The best thing that happened after being diagnosed was finding the PIEN." Linda's hobby is graphic arts and she is the proud grandmother of 1-year-old Skyler.

WILLIAM MICHEAL (BILL) HARRINGTON, 45, lives on Vancouver Island off the coast of British Columbia, Canada, and was diagnosed 16 years ago. His works have appeared in PD newsletters in the United States, England, Australia, and Canada. Two books, *dream warrior*, a collection of his poetry, and an art book, combining his prose with art by Lillian Dyck, will be published in 2001. Bill is father of "two fine sons, Adam, 22, and Lee, 19."

Rick Hermann, 50, works for an engineering society as a book publisher, is married to Lee, and has a teenage son, Eli. Rick bicycles the 4 miles to work every day, rain or shine. He was diagnosed with Parkinson's in January 1998.

TIM HODGENS, PH.D., is a psychologist in private practice in Westborough, Massachusetts. His professional interests include stress management and its influence on Parkinson's disease.

WILL JOHNSTON, PH.D., taught economics, finance, and risk management at a number of universities. He first experienced PD symptoms at age 39, but was not correctly diagnosed until he was 58. Will, now 68, serves as president of the DelMarVa Chapter of APDA, publishes *The Parkinson's Newsletter*, participates in PD research, and with his wife, Mary Margaret, is involved in volunteer activities in Salisbury, Maryland.

CELIA JONES immigrated to Melbourne, Australia, in 1972 from Berkeley, California. She was a high school teacher/librarian when she was diagnosed at age 41, and retired 9 years later due to PD. She is active in Young Parkinson's support groups, gives speeches for the newly diagnosed, and works with the Young Parkinson's Housing Project.

IDA KAMPHUIS is a retired psychologist and psychotherapist from the Netherlands who was diagnosed in 1984, at the age of 40. She writes, "I had to stop working immediately after being diagnosed, and that was devastating. For some years I have been in very bad shape, but a pallidotomy has kind of saved me." She and her husband, parents of two grown children, are both ferocious readers and are now looking forward to traveling in southern Europe.

DAVID LANGRIDGE of the United Kingdom says, "When I was first diagnosed 8 years ago, I bought my first computer and learned word processing, as I knew my handwriting would suffer. Little did I realize then what a boon the growth of the Internet would bring to disablement...I have learned and shared so much about Parkinson's from this medium. I firmly believe that Parkinson's can be a gateway to new interests and, contrary to conventional medical science, have faith that this disease is not forever."

BARBARA MALLUT of Southern California writes, "I see myself evolving, but at the same time, PD is forcing me to narrow my world. I tend to take life's side streets now instead of heading for life's freeways. Once-upon-a-time I'd have been bored to tears traveling through life in the 'slow lane,' but now I find there are tons of interesting things as well as interesting people lining those little offbeat roads. I've come to know and enjoy them as they add to my life in many ways."

ROBERT A. (BOB) MARTONE is a retired CPA, oil company executive, and caregiver for his wife, NANCY, who has had PD for 26 years. They have been married for the past 36 years. Bob is active on several charitable foundation boards and is past President of the Houston Area Parkinson Society.

CHARLES MEYER, 56, is a psychiatrist but is no longer practicing. Born in Philadelphia, Pennsylvania, he now lives in Madison, Wisconsin, with his wife, Ellen. He developed Parkinson's about 12 years ago. Ellen and Charlie have three grown children (the youngest a senior in college) and one grandchild.

SONIA NIELSEN is from Denmark. She writes, "I'm living with my disease and not for it. I choose every day that this day will be a special good day. It's a bad disease to live with, but it has good side effects as well—it has given me a new and very exciting life."

SANDRA NORRIS lives in North Carolina and has battled with PD since she was 20 (nearly 20 years ago). Sandra believes her strength comes from her faith in God, family, and friends. A whole new world was opened to her when she became a participant in the online mailing list Parkinson's Information Exchange Network.

RICHARD L. PIKUNIS, JR., was 27 when he was diagnosed in 1996. He is now an attorney, emphasizing criminal defense, and resides in New Jersey with his wife, Lynn, and two young sons, Justin and Alex. He writes, "I am determined to fight until a cure for PD is a reality, not only for myself, but also for my children. I love them so much and can't see myself not being there for them in every way."

JOHN QVIST, 32, was also diagnosed at age 27. He is a Web developer and project coordinator at the National Board for Higher Education in Sweden. Before Parkinson's, John took part in ballroom dancing, martial arts, and rock climbing. He still enjoys working out, theater and cinema, and backpacking.

BARB RAGER, 54, is a retired teacher from Ottawa, Ontario. She writes, "The stages of grieving bound around a family like a three-legged dog. Just as one person is coming up from the sense of the devastation wrought by this disease, another is going down. With my own two boys gone, now men and launched into their own vital lives, my husband and I must look honestly at each other and revisit our dreams. And, when that is done, we must revisit them again. Life doesn't end with Parkinson's. Many things do end with it, it is true. But while there is still life, there is life!"

SUSAN REESE, a registered nurse and clinical social worker, is the Coordinator of both the APDA Illinois/Indiana Regional Parkinson's Information & Referral Center and the APDA National Young-Onset Center. Susan is a frequent lecturer on various aspects of coping with Parkinson's disease and has been interviewed on the NBC *Today Show* and other national television programs.

ALAN RICHARDS, from London, Ontario, Canada, was a newspaper copy editor for more than 30 years. He took an early retirement shortly after his wife, Judith's, diagnosis and now works with the Young-Onset Connection support group in London and volunteers at the Parkinson Society Canada/Société Parkinson Canada's regional office. His hobbies include genealogy and photography.

JUDITH RICHARDS was a hospital switchboard supervisor when Parkinson's arrived and is now on long-term disability. She has been an active member of the Parkinsn List, coleader of the Parkinson's Young-Onset Connection in London, and has lectured to Parkinson's support groups throughout western Ontario. Judith's hobbies are gardening, decorating, crafts, and cooking. Alan and Judith have four grown children.

CHRIS ROBIE of Melbourne, Australia, was diagnosed at age 40 in 1989. He is active in the Young Parkinson Housing Project, telelink, bicycle riding, and addressing the needs of Young Parkies who have been deserted or are single. Chris's ambition is to meet Michael J. Fox.

JANE ROSS of Oregon says, "I have found a second family that I love on the Internet. We are linked together with a common bond of hope and fear while we fight Parkinson's disease."

ANNE RUTHERFORD of Newfoundland, Canada, was diagnosed in 1980 at age 39 and is the third generation in her family to have PD. Anne was a founding member and first president of Newfoundland and Labrador Chapter of the Parkinson Society Canada/Société Parkinson Canada and is editor of *Newfoundland Parkinson News*. Anne underwent a pallidotomy in April 1996, with good but temporary results. She says, "I've had to give up many interests due to PD, but I still have my garden."

BARBARA SCHIRLOFF's brother Ron was diagnosed in 1994 at age 50. Ron is still employed but "in the closet" at work. Barb, who is from New Jersey, became active in Parkinson's advocacy in 1995, and it is her "chief outside interest, because the cure seems so close."

JIM SLATTERY was diagnosed in 1984 at age 45. After being discharged by his employer, the State Public Service of New South Wales, Australia, in 1986, he began a new career as a lecturer in information technology at the local campus of the department of technical and further education, which he continued to do for 8 years. While there, he became acquainted with Dr. Jim Selby, who was interested in using computers as recovery therapy for stroke patients. By coincidence, Dr. Selby later contracted PD and again sought Jim out to assist, this time in a study of Parkinsonians and caregivers.

JOAN SNYDER, 49, lives in Chillicothe, Illinois, with her husband, Stan, and children, Allison, 13, and Mitchell, 11. Diagnosed when she was 38, Joan underwent two pallidotomies. She is creative communications director for the Parkinson's Alliance; works with researchers at the University of Illinois School of Medicine, providing input from the point of view of the PD patient; and coedited *Voices from the Parking Lot.*

IVAN MFOWETHU SUZMAN, 51, is an anthropologist who grew up in Providence, Rhode Island, and now lives in Portland, Maine. In the 1970s, he traveled to Africa, where his work included descriptions of early human fossil discoveries from Ethiopia, Kenya, Tanzania, and South Africa. He later taught at the University of Minnesota Medical School and Bowdoin College in Maine. Parkinson's has restricted his career since the early 1990s, but he remains active as an advocate for PD research funding and awareness. He also appears regularly on local stage and radio.

JOHN TESTA, from Rochester, New York, was 45 years old when he was diagnosed 6 years ago. John is a Vietnam-era Air Force veteran, has a B.A. in history, and works in production and inventory management.

DONNA TESTA, John's wife, who is a nurse and a professional clown, often lectures on PD in their community. Donna and John created an international "Ball of String Project" in 1997 to raise PD awareness.

PHIL TOMPKINS of Amherst, Massachusetts, was diagnosed at the age of 51. After 9 years with PD, he retired from his career as a computer programmer due to his increasingly erratic response to levodopa, dyskinesia, fatigue, and insomnia. Phil has since put his computer skills to good use as creator and webmaster of *Index to Parkinson's Disease Information on the Internet* (http://www.pdindex.org).

MARGARET TUCHMAN was born in Budapest, Hungary, and immigrated to the United States with her parents after the Hungarian revolution in 1956. Her diagnosis of Parkinson's came in 1981. As a founding member of the Parkinson Alliance, she now dedicates her time to raising money for research. The Internet has also provided her with an outlet for one of her lifelong passions—creating Habitat for Horses, a sanctuary for abused and unwanted horses. She spends hours raising funds for equine-assisted therapy programs that help people who are emotionally, mentally, and physically challenged.

GAIL VASS's sister EDNA EARLE was diagnosed with PD at the age of 49.

RITA WEEKS, 56, enjoys sewing and gardening. She was diagnosed with Parkinson's when she was in her early 40s. Rita and her husband, Don, live in Lincoln, Nebraska. They have four grown children and two grandchildren.

DIETMAR WESSEL, age 46, lives near Frankfurt, Germany, and was diagnosed at the age of 34. Married with two children, he was project manager for development aid projects of the United Nations and a German development bank. PD forced him to retire in 1999. Dietmar created the German-speaking PD mailing list DEUPARK and is the patient representative in a European Commission financed research project on virtual reality walking aids for PD patients, and telerehabilitation through videoconferencing.

MARY YOST is a mother, amateur musician, and a recently retired university administrator from Los Angeles, California. Since her diagnosis at age 42, she has been involved with Parkinson's support groups and political advocacy. Her interest in tai chi for PWP led to a pilot study at the University of Southern California. In 2000, she cofounded Team Parkinson, an official charity for the L.A. Marathon, and with her nephew, "Coach T," completed the 26.2-mile course in 9 hours and 18 minutes.

Ideas for Advocates

BY JEANETTE FUHR

During the collaboration on and writing of *When Parkinson's Strikes Early*, I volunteered as group cheerleader. My adopted role was to encourage, to suggest, and to comment on the emerging "baby." As the "godmother" to this creation, I began to realize that when people find they have a chronic, incurable disease, there is a natural desire "to do something" to help or to change the situation. This desire is present in people diagnosed with any serious disease, be it Parkinson's, cancer, diabetes, or other illnesses.

In my own life with Parkinson's, my first action was to read material about the disease. An article authored by Barb in the newsletter of the Parkinson Association of Greater Kansas City caught my eye, and as a result of reading that article I sent my first ever e-mail asking Barb about support from others with Parkinson's. I found "my voice" as I joined PIEN and started asking questions, speaking boldly to medical professionals treating me for PD symptoms, and even asking friends, family, and church family to help me be heard. Both Barb and Linda agreed that I was evolving into a grassroots advocate for Parkinson's disease. My metamorphosis from a quiet, shy, retiring woman into a vocal, brave, outspoken woman has been an interesting process.

In this section, I have compiled a number of actions anyone reading this book can try in response to the question "what can I do about Parkinson's disease?"

These are ideas I have implemented myself, and actions undertaken by other list members, to raise awareness of PD or to raise funds for focused research into its causes, treatments, and cure.

Some of these are simple and inexpensive and can be done from your home or office. Others are more complicated, involve some expense, and require publicity and openness.

It is my hope that the questing person will read these suggestions and react by saying, "Yes, I *will* do that; it's a positive action that will help those who have Parkinson's disease." In addition, I hope that persons experiencing similar extreme challenges from other conditions or diseases will be exposed to and learn from this grassroots advocacy model.

To-Do List

(See the resource guide, Appendix 2, for more information on starred items.)

1. Write letters to or call your elected officials asking for funding to support focused Parkinson's research at the National Institutes of Health (NIH) or your own government's medical-research agency.

2. Write letters to the editors of newspapers and magazines, especially when the publications have printed articles about Michael J. Fox, Muhammad Ali, or others with Parkinson's.

3. Write or call to thank the media when programs or news stories feature Parkinson's legislation, treatments, etc., and offer to provide follow-up information.

4. Circulate and get signatures on petitions from people in groups you belong to or have the opportunity to visit, requesting funding appropriations from Congress for focused Parkinson's research at NIH.

5. Raise awareness by asking local groups to support April as Parkinson's Awareness Month. To help increase publicity, you might ask your mayor, your governor, or the president of your country to sign a proclamation designating April as Parkinson's Awareness Month. Pose with the official and your group for a photo for the media.

6. ★ Join or start a support group for Parkinson's patients, caregivers, and friends.

7. Suggest and plan awareness campaigns for Parkinson's.

8. ★ Write news releases about donations to the research seed-money campaign of the Parkinson's Alliance.

9. Try something like Bowling for Parkinson's, a successful fund-raiser run by Kees Paap in his community.

10. Take a piggy bank to places you normally go and ask for donations for Parkinson's research, following the example of Hilary Blue and her piggy bank, named Porquina.

11. ★ Order and sell any type of Parkinson's pin (for example, tulip pins are available from the Parkinson Society Canada/ Société Parkinson Canada).

12. ★ Distribute pamphlets and information sheets from local or national PD organizations at health fairs held at hospitals, senior centers, schools, etc.

13. Seek grants from private and public health organizations to fund the dissemination of information via phone voicemail, similar to the County Connection Line of Grundy County, Missouri, which has established voicemail for health and public-service information.

14. ★ Raise money for research by obtaining pledges and participating in the NYC Unity Walk, Team Parkinson at the Los Angeles Marathon, or other PD walks—or organize your own walk or run.

15. Design and market Parkinson's-awareness T-shirts, and donate the proceeds for research and care.

16. ★ Tell your own or your friend's or family member's story about life with Parkinson's on a member page of the PWP Web ring, at <http://www.newcountry.nu/pd/members/index.htm>.

17. Allow others to see the person behind the "mask": volunteer to be a guest speaker and to inform others about Parkinson's.

18. ★ Join an Internet discussion group or chat room.

19. Print business cards with the name, meeting place, and time of your support group. Give them to PWPs or to others who may know PWPs, and invite them to join.

20. Keep up your social and recreational activities even when it would be easier to "just stay home."

21. Form liaisons with your peers at work, in community groups, and with the parents and teachers of your children's friends, allowing you remain active in spite of the limitations that Parkinson's may cause.

22. Be an advocate for others who are challenged by any limitation by insisting that all people be given the opportunity to participate.

23. Rejoice each day, for there is something good in each day.

24. Exercise your mind, your body, and your options regularly.

25. Teach others that tolerance and patience are two important traits to cultivate. For example, if individuals seem impatient with you, simply explain, "Please be patient, I'm doing the best I can with Parkinson's."

26. Think positively and act accordingly.

27. Accept the things you cannot change, change the things you can, and ask for the wisdom to know the difference (from the serenity prayer).

28. Organize and hold a flea market or garage sale to raise funds for and awareness of Parkinson's disease.

29. Involve student groups from preschool through college in walk-a-thons, health fairs, and nursing-home projects to raise awareness and funds for Parkinson's patients and research.

30. Increase your aerobic activities (walking, jogging, or other aerobic activities) to improve your health.

31. Bend, stretch, and lift weights to increase your flexibility and strength and thus improve your ability to do some or all of these activities.

32. ★★★ Buy copies of this book for gifts. Authors' royalties from its sale go to Parkinson's research.

appendix 2

A Selective Resource Guide to Parkinson's Disease Information

The following books, videos, websites, and other Internet resources have been recommended by members of the Parkinson's Information Exchange Network:

Books, Newsletters, and Videos

Biziere, Kathleen E., and Matthias C. Kurth. *Living with Parkinson's Disease*. New York: Demos Vermande, 1997.

Carlton, Lucille. *Sex, Love and Chronic Illness*. Miami, FL: National Parkinson Foundation, 1994. (May be ordered from NPF by calling (800) 327-4545.)

Coleman, Barbara, and Barry Green, eds. *The Parkinson Predicament and a Spoonful of Sugar: My Life with Parkinson's Disease*. Tyler, TX: Parkinsonian Publications, 1997.

Cote, Lucian, et al. *Parkinson's Disease and Quality of Life*. New York: Haworth Press, 2000.

Cram, David L. *Understanding Parkinson's Disease: A Self-Help Guide*. Omaha, NE: Addicus Books, 1999.

Duvoisin, Roger C., and Jacob I. Sage. *Parkinson's Disease: A Guide for Patient and Family*. Philadelphia, PA: Lippincott-Williams & Wilkins, 1995.

Grady-Fitchell, Joan. *Flying Lessons: On the Wings of Parkinson's Disease*. New York: Forge Press, 1998.

Graham, Joy. *Lost Voices: Hospitalisation—Potential Minefields in Parkinson's Disease*. This video was created to train nurses and other health-care personnel about possible problems and dangers facing hospitalized PWP. (Contact the publisher to order: Parkinson's Association of WA, ADA House, 54-58 Havelock St., PO Box 910, West Perth 6872, Australia or call: 08 9322 9322.)

Greene, Dennis, Joan Blessington Snyder, and Craig L. Kendall, eds. *Voices from the Parking Lot: Parkinson's Insights and Perspectives*. Princeton, NJ: The Parkinson's Alliance, 2000. (Order from The Parkinson's Alliance, 211 College Rd. East, Princeton, NJ 08540 or call (800) 579-8440.)

Grimes, J. David, and David A. Grimes. *Parkinson's: One Step at a Time: Problems and Answers for Patients and Health Professionals*. Third ed. Ottawa, Canada: Parkinson's Society of Ottawa, 1999. (May be ordered from the Parkinson's Society by calling (613) 722-9238.)

Hauser, Robert, Theresa Zesiewicz, and Abraham Lieberman. *Parkinson's Disease*. Coral Springs, FL: Merit Publishing, 2000.

Holden, Kathrynne. *Eat Well, Stay Well with Parkinson's Disease: A Nutrition Handbook for People with Parkinson's*. Fort Collins, CO: Five Star Living, 2000.

———. *Eat Well, Stay Well with Parkinson's Disease: A Nutrition Handbook for People with Parkinson's*. Australian edition, edited by Linley Boulden. West Perth, Australia: The Parkinson's Association of Western Australia Inc., 1999. (To order: contact The Parkinson's Association of Western Australia, PO Box 910, West Perth, WA 6872, Australia.)

———. *Parkinson's Disease—Guidelines for Medical Nutrition Therapy: A Manual for Nutrition Professionals*. Fort Collins, CO: Five Star Living, 2000. (May be ordered by calling (877) 565-2665.)

———. *Parkinson's Disease and Constipation* (cassette and booklet for individual and group use). Fort Collins, CO: Five Star Living, 2000.

Hutton, J. Thomas, and Raye Lynn Dippel. *Caring for the Parkinson Patient*. Amherst, NY: Prometheus Books, 1999.

Kondracke, Morton. *Saving Millie: Love, Politics and Parkinson's Disease*. New York: Public Affairs, 2001.

Landau, Elaine. *Parkinson's Disease* (young adult book). New York: Franklin Watts, 1999.

Langston, J. William. *The Case of the Frozen Addicts*. New York: Vintage Books, 1996.

Lieberman, Abraham. *Parkinson's Disease: The Complete Guide for Patients and Caregivers*. New York: Simon & Schuster, 1993.

———. *Shaking Up Parkinson's Disease: Fighting Like a Tiger, Thinking Like a Fox*. Jones and Bartlett, 2001.

Mark, Margery, and Jacob Sage, eds. *Young Parkinson's Handbook: A Guide for Patients and Their Families*. Staten Island, NY: American Parkinson Disease Association, 2000.

Mcenaney, Tena Parisoff. *In Search of a Champion: The Early Onset Parkinson's Project*. Video, 30 minutes in color. St. Joseph, MO: Visual Logic, 2000. Distributed by Parkinson Association of Greater Kansas City, 7808 Foster, Overland Park, KS 66204-2955. To order, call (913) 341-8828, fax (913) 341-8885, or e-mail pagkc@aol.com.

Morgan, Eric R. *Defending Against the Enemy: Coping with Parkinson's Disease*. Fort Bragg, CA: QED Press, 1997.

My Spirit Still Sings. Video produced by The Young Parkinson's Housing Project in Australia, provides an inside, moving look at the housing and care challenges faced by young-onset Parkinson's sufferers (13 min.). (To order: contact Young Parkinson's Housing Incorporated, PO Box 134, Darling, Victoria, Australia 3145.)

The Parkinson Education Team Video. The Parkinson Education Team, consisting of three patients and their caregivers, describes the disease, how it affects the body and manifests itself in the various symptoms, and how each team member reacted to the first diagnosis of Parkinson's. A teaching tool for patients, family members, and health-care staff, the video is priced at $30 for individuals and $100 for corporations. To order, contact Young-Onset and Care Partner Support Group, Denver, CO, by calling (303) 830-1839 or e-mail ParRockies@aol.com.

Parkinson's Disease—Early Onset Video. (Speaking from Experience series) Produced with advice from Parkinson's Victoria, the video presents commentary from two single and two partnered younger Parkinsonians about their reactions to their diagnosis and the coping strategies they have developed. (To order: contact TRIBAL, 50 Rouse St., Port Melbourne, Melbourne, VIC 3207, Australia or call: (03) 9645 2222.)

Parkinsonian People: an independent tabloid newspaper by and for Parkinsonians. Tyler, TX: Parkinsonian Publications. Quarterly. To subscribe: Contact Barry Green, editor, 4801 Richmond Rd., Tyler, TX 75703 or by calling (903) 509-0054.

Quist, Jan. *My Mommy Has PD...but It's OK!* (children's book). Glenview, IL: American Parkinson Disease Association Young-Onset Information and Referral Center, 2001. This book is available through the Center at 2100 Pfingsten Rd., Glenview, IL 60025 or by calling (800) 223-9776.

The Uninvited Guest: Young-Onset Parkinson's Disease. Video recording produced by YAPP&Rs (Young Alert Parkinson's Partners & Relatives), Great Britain. It uses a combination of drama and real-life interviews to provide an insight into living with PD as a young person and to offer hope by highlighting the support provided by the United Kingdom's Parkinson's Disease Society and its special-interest group, YAPP&Rs, for younger people with PD. (To order: contact PDS Sales Ltd., Westerfield Business Centre, Main Rd., Westerfield, Ipswich, Suffolk, UK, IP6 9AB or phone 0044-1473-212115.)

Weiner, William J., Lisa M. Shulman, and Anthony E. Lang. *Parkinson's Disease: A Complete Guide for Patients and Families.* Baltimore, MD: Johns Hopkins University Press, 2001.

Parkinson's Disease on the World Wide Web

There are hundreds of websites about PD. The following are highly recommended by members of the PIEN list for being informative, accurate, and up to date. Each category is in alphabetical order. Also see "Parkinson's Organizations Worldwide," below. Many of these organizations maintain excellent websites. The URLs or Internet addresses indicated are active as of June 2001, but, like everything on the Internet, are subject to change.

Subject Directories and Indexes to PD Websites: Good Places to Start

Internet subject directories and indexes provide linked listings of websites, arranged by subject matter. Their compilers often evaluate the sites for usefulness, accuracy, and timeliness before including them, and review them periodically.

Ask NOAH (New York Online Access to Health—Parkinson's Disease)
http://www.noah-health.org/english/illness/neuro/parkin.html

Index to Parkinson's Disease Information on the Internet
Very comprehensive and well indexed. Compiled by Phil Tompkins, PIEN list member.
http://www.pdindex.org

Parkinson's Web—Massachusetts General Hospital
http://pdweb.mgh.harvard.edu/

PIENO—Parkinsons Information Exchange Network Online

The official website of the PIEN (Parkinsn List) was created and is maintained by list member John Cottingham. It consists of a number of treasures, including:

Parkinsn List Messages Online provides access to the most recent 500 messages to the PIEN mailing list; plus links to other PD information; a message board; access to the list's complete, searchable archives; and subscription options.

http://www.parkinsons-information-exchange-network-online.com/parkmail/maillist.html

The Parkinsn List Drug Database cites over 140 drugs that Parkinson's patients might encounter and details the possible side effects and contraindications of each. Drugs that the Parkinson's patient should avoid postoperatively are also detailed.

http://www.parkinsons-information-exchange-network-online.com/drugdb/drugdb.html

The Parkinsn Current Topics Archive Treasures provides the full text of important articles and studies on Parkinson's and discussions on common questions.

http://www.parkinsons-information-exchange-network-online.com/

Parkinsn List Archives is a searchable database of all messages to the Parkinsn List, 1993–present. It is maintained by list member Simon Coles.

http://parkinsn.coles.org.uk/

Recommended Websites on Young-Onset Parkinson's Disease

American Parkinson Disease Association Young Parkinson's Information & Referral Center

Provides very useful information about PD and services available through the center, online articles from the *Young Parkinson's Newsletter*, and links to other PD resources.

http://members.aol.com/apdaypd/young/index.html

Awakenings Website

"Young Onset Parkinson's Disease" and "Attitude in PD: A Personal Perspective" are two excellent articles by Emma Bennion, of YAPP&Rs, an organization for young-onset PWPs in Great

Britain. Available online at:
http://www.parkinsonsdisease.com/lwp/ygonset.htm

Young Parkinson's Handbook

Web version of the guide published by the American Parkinson Disease Association (see "Books and Videos," above). Covers topics such as symptoms, medications, nutrition, the workplace, financial issues, families, sexuality, and relationships. Available online at:

http://neuro-chief-e.mgh.harvard.edu/parkinsonsweb/Main/YOPD_ Handbook/YOPD_TOC.html#TOC

Especially Recommended for the Newly Diagnosed

The Newly Diagnosed

From the website of SPRING (Special Parkinson's Research Interest Group), part of the Parkinson's Disease Society of the UK.

http://spring.parkinsons.org.uk/spnewly.htm

The Newly Diagnosed

Helpful facts and information from the Parkinson Society Canada/Société Parkinson Canada.

http://parkinson.ca/pd/nd.html

Parkinson's Facts

Valuable information from the National Parkinson's Foundation.

http://www.parkinson.org/eduindex.htm

Other PIEN-Recommended Websites

Awakenings

International in scope, this site provides current news, treatments, research, links to PD organizations and support groups around the world.

http://www.parkinsonsdisease.com

CenterWatch Clinical Trials Listing Service

An international listing of industry- and government-sponsored clinical trials that are actively recruiting patients. Search by therapeutic area and geographic region. Sign up for e-mail notification of new trials.

http://www.centerwatch.com/main.htm

Clinical Trials

Lists currently recruiting clinical trials from the National Institutes of Health. Search on "Parkinson."

http://clinicaltrials.gov/ct/gui

Diagnostic Criteria for PD

From *Archives of Neurology* (online). Outlines the clinical signs neurologists look for in diagnosing PD.

http://archneur.ama-assn.org/issues/v56n1/rfull/nsa7701.html

James: A Site About Parkinson's

PIEN list member Simon Cole's website; a valuable source about the international online PD community, plus other informative links.

http://james.parkinsons.org.uk/

Medscape Neurology Home Page

The targeted audience is medical practitioners, but there is a wealth of information here for the informed patient as well. The latest research findings, news, conference reports, selected journal articles, resources for patients, and more. Requires free registration.

http://www.medscape.com/Home/Topics/Neurology/Neurology.html

Morris K. Udall Home Page

From the University of Arizona Library. Learn more about Congressman "Mo" Udall, an inspiration to many PWPs, through this fascinating archive of his speeches, publications, and other documents.

http://dizzy.library.arizona.edu/branches/spc/udall/homepage.html

National Institute of Neurological Disorders and Stroke, National Institutes of Health

A good source for up-to-date information, U.S. government-funded research, and other medical news.

http://www.ninds.nih.gov/

NINDS Parkinson's Disease Research Web

http://www.ninds.nih.gov/parkinsonsweb

National Parkinson's Foundation Online Publications

A listing of NPF's publications is at:

http://www.parkinson.org/onlinpub.htm

The following publications from this excellent and comprehensive collection have received rave reviews:

▶ Adjustment, Adaptation, and Accommodation: Psychosocial Approaches to Living with Parkinson's Disease

▶ Parkinson's Disease: Fitness Counts

- ▶ Parkinson's Disease: Medications
- ▶ Parkinson's Disease: Nutrition Matters (NPF Special Edition: excerpts from Kathrynne Holden's book, *Eat Well, Stay Well with Parkinson's Disease*; see "Books and Videos," above)
- ▶ Parkinson's Disease: Speaking Out, by National Parkinson Foundation Speech Team

Northwest Parkinson's Foundation Website

This regional PD organization's site wins honors; it is always very informative and up to date, with research news, PD links, articles, *Parkinson's Post* newsletter, frequently asked questions, and other resources.

http://www.nwpf.org/

Quality, Delivery, and Access to Parkinson's Care

A Web-based public-health research and advocacy program of the Parkinson's Disease Foundation, directed by PIEN list member Dr. Perry Cohen.

http://www.parkinsonscare.org

Disability Information

APDA Young Parkinson's Information and Referral Center: Online Articles on Disability:

Applying for Disability—Fall/ Winter 1997

Employment: What Does The Americans With Disabilities Act Mean To You?—Summer 2000

Helpful Social Security Disability Resources—Summer/Fall 1998

http://members.aol.com/apdaypd/young/index.html

JAN on the Web: Job Accommodations Network

An international toll-free consulting service that provides information about job accommodations and the employability of people with disabilities.

http://www.jan.wvu.edu/

JAN: SOAR (Searchable Online Accommodations Database) provides accommodation options for persons with disabilities in the workplace.

http://www.jan.wvu.edu/soar/index.html

SEE: **Accommodating Parkinson's Disease** for possible solutions and ideas for workplace problems of PWP:

http://www.jan.wvu.edu/media/PD.html

JAN also provides extensive links to web resources on the Americans with Disabilities Act:

http://jan.wvu.edu/links/adalinks.htm

Parkinsn (PIEN Website) Current Topics:
What Parkinsonians Should Know About Social Security
Disability

http://www.parkinsons-information-exchange-network-online.com/archive/011.html

Disability Evaluation under Social Security

Presents the rules the Social Security Administration uses to evaluate disabilities.

http://www.parkinsons-information-exchange-network-online.com/archive/012.html

Parkinson's Disease and Social Security Disability Insurance (SSDI)

Maintained and compiled by PIEN list member Greg Sterling, this site contains information on eligibility, applying, the appeals process, sample letters, legal issues, links to Social Security Administration sites, and other helpful Web links.

http://pd_ssdi.homestead.com/ssdi.html

Web Resources for Advocates

Congress.org

Locate elected officials by zip codes, research their voting record, send them an e-mail message, and find information on current issues.

http://congress.org/

Consortium for Citizens with Disabilities

"A coalition of approximately 100 national disability organizations working together to advocate for national public policy that ensures the self-determination, independence, empowerment, integration, and inclusion of children and adults with disabilities in all aspects of society."

http://www.c-c-d.org/index.htm

Families USA: the Voice for Health Care Consumers

Provides information on and advocates for health insurance coverage for all children, the disabled and the working poor, improving Medicaid and Medicare, long-term care, disability rights and other health policy issues.

http://www.familiesusa.org/

Kaisernetwork:

Provides information and analysis on federal and state level health policy issues. Reports are updated daily.

http://www.kaisernetwork.org/

Thomas: Legislative information on the Internet (in the spirit on Thomas Jefferson).

Follow a bill's progress through Congress, read comments, testimonies and speeches, find voting schedules and records, link to other political websites, and more.

http://thomas.loc.gov

People with Parkinson's in Cyberspace: Mailing Lists, Chat Rooms, Web Forums

Mailing Lists

A mailing list is a list of e-mail addresses identified by a single name, such as parkinsn@listserv.utoronto.ca. When an e-mail message is sent to the mailing-list name, it is automatically forwarded to all the addresses in the list. Mailing lists may be dedicated to specific subjects, such as the PD-oriented lists below. All require free subscriptions.

Directory of Worldwide Mailing Lists

Links to the following PD mailing lists from around the world, and instructions for subscribing to them, can be found at Simon Coles's website:

http://james.parkinsons.org.uk/community.htm

PARKINSN LIST, also called **PIEN** (Parkinson Information and Exchange Network).

An English-language international mailing list, with over 2,000 subscribers representing 37 nations. To subscribe, send an e-mail message to:

listserv@listsev.utoronto.ca

In the body of the message type: SUBSCRIBE PARKINSN [YOUR FIRST NAME] [YOUR LAST NAME]

CARE (Caregivers Are Really Essential)

A sublist of PIEN especially for PD caregivers (CGs). List owner Camilla Flintermann writes: "The need for such a list was evident from feelings expressed on the PD list that there were times when CGs needed to be able to "let off steam" in a place where this would not upset care partners (CPs). Some of us have caregiver support groups, where we can safely express feelings, get practical support, and share experiences—others do not. The CARE list serves this need, but DOES NOT shut off participation by CGs on the main list." Caregivers who wish to join should e-mail Camilla Flintermann for instructions, as this is a closed list: flintepc@muohio.edu.

PDKIDS

Membership in PDKIDS is for children only. The following description is by Susan Reese, R.N., LCSW, American Parkinson Disease Association Young-Onset Information and Referral Center:

The American Parkinson Disease Association Young Parkinson's Information and Referral Center (http://members.aol.com/apdaypd/young/index.html) has created PDKIDS, an e-mail discussion list for children who are living in a family or love someone affected by Parkinson's disease.

Parkinson's disease is a family affair. Even young children are affected when someone they love is not functioning in his or her "normal" ways. PDKIDS is a forum for children (through teenage years) who live with or love someone with Parkinson's disease. Through this Internet program, PDKIDS offers children a place to get to know others like themselves who are in similar circumstances and have similar concerns. By joining PDKIDS, children can "talk" to each other in confidence (to the extent that an Internet list will allow) and discuss anything they wish about how PD affects them.

This is a free program for any child under 18 years of age.

To join, kids simply send an e-mail to: join-pdkids@lyris.coles.org.uk.

You will then receive a welcome message with instructions about how to use PDKIDS.

When you reply to an e-mail, your response will go directly to the PDKIDS list, not to an individual member.

There will be a "light adult presence" on the list, serving to provide technical guidance and to ensure that the conversation remains constructive.

This "presence" will be provided by Susan Reese, R.N., LCSW, Coordinator of the APDA Young Parkinson's Information and

Referral Center, and by Simon Coles, co-owner of the list, and himself an adult PD kid.

For more information, call the APDA Young-Onset Center at (800) 223-9776.

PDNEWS

The following description is by Simon Coles:

PDNEWS is an announcement list for people with Parkinson's, their families and caregivers, health-care professionals, and other people with an interest in Parkinson's disease matters. Traffic is low, typically one or two articles a week, with articles covering new resources and events, as well as articles of particular interest from other Parkinson's-related mailing lists.

PDNEWS is for people who want to remain informed of developments in the Parkinson's disease world, without having to participate in the main (high-volume) PIEN list.

Archives of the list and other information is available at:

http://www.pdnews.org/pdnews.htm

To subscribe to PDNEWS, use the web interface at:

http://lists.nipltd.com/cgi-bin/lyris.pl?join=pdnews

Or, send a regular e-mail message (content doesn't matter) to:

join-pdnews@lyris.coles.org.uk

PDUK

A mailing list for United Kingdom–specific Parkinson's issues.
Archives of the list and other information are available at:

http://www.coles.org.uk/Current_Projects/Lists/pduk.htm

A Web interface to the mailing list can be used to subscribe, unsubscribe, view the list archives, etc., and is found at:

http://lists.nipltd.com/cgi-bin/lyris.pl?enter=pduk

Or, subscribe to PDUK by sending an e-mail message to:

join-pduk@lyris.coles.org.uk

Or, write to list owner Simon Coles at: simon@nipltd.com

BELGAPARK

The Belgian Parkinson's list (in French, Flemish, English, German, and Spanish). Contact list owner Martine Semal by e-mail at: m_semal@hotmail.com

Information is available at:

http://www.coles.org.uk/Current_Projects/Lists/belgapark.htm

DEUPARK

A German-speaking list about Parkinson's. For information, contact the owners: Dietmar Wessel by e-mail at: DietmarW@compuserve.com or Simon Coles at: simon@nipltd.com

Information is also available on the Web at: http://www.coles.org.uk/Current_Projects/Lists/deupark.htm

NEDERPARK

The Dutch-language PD list. More information can be found at: http://people.zeelandnet.nl/genugten/nederprk.htm

Or, e-mail list owner Hans van der Genugten at: genugten@zeelandnet.nl

The following two Dutch-language mailing lists are also under Hans's direction:

MANTELPARK

The Dutch-language list for caregivers. Information is available at: http://people.zeelandnet.nl/genugten/mantlprk.htm

PARKJEUGD

A discussion list for children whose parents or other family members have Parkinson's. To learn more, see: http://people.zeelandnet.nl/genugten/prkjeugd.htm

PARKINSON

A mailing list for speakers of Spanish. Archives are available at: http://listserv.rediris.es/archives/parkinson.html

For more information, contact the list owner at: PARKINSON-request@LISTSERV.REDIRIS.ES

To subscribe, send an e-mail to: LISTSERV@LISTSERV.REDIRIS.ES with the command: SUBSCRIBE PARKINSON

PARKLISTE

An international French-speaking list. The Parkliste website is at: http://www.parkliste.org/

For more information, contact Bernard Joly, Président de Parkliste, by e-mail at: parkliste.parkinson@wanadoo.fr

Yngre Parkinson

Swedish Young Parkinsons. Contact list owner Paul Petersson for information at: paul.r.petersson@telia.com

Chat Rooms

Chat rooms are websites that allow online, real-time discussions to take place between any number of individuals. Participants may have to register for a password first and then log into a particular chat room, or the discussion may be open to anyone entering that site at the time. Some chat room sites are always open for anyone who "drops" in; others are online at only specified times.

PWP Dumpster Gang Community
Website and chat room at:
http://anexa.com/pwp/index.lhtml

People Living with Parkinson's Chat Room (on YAHOO)
http://clubs.yahoo.com/clubs/plwp

Web Forums

Web forums allow participants with common interests to post and read open messages. Forums are sometimes called discussion or bulletin boards. They usually don't require subscriptions and are open for all.

PWP Dumpster Gang Community
Public discussion board at:
http://anexa.com/pwp/forums/publicForum.lhtml

Brain Talk Community
This forum from Massachusetts General Hospital hosts two PD
    forums: Parkinson's Disease Forum and PLWP (People Living
    with Parkinson's) Organization Forum. Both are accessible from:
http://neuro-mancer.mgh.harvard.edu/cgi-bin/Ultimate.cgi

National Parkinson Foundation Discussion Forums
The Parkinson's disease forum is accessible through:
http://www.parkinson.org/shell/lyris.pl

Additional chat rooms and forums can be found on the Yahoo Clubs for Parkinson's Disease website:
    http://dir.clubs.yahoo.com/Health__Wellness/Support/Illnesses/Parkinson_s_Disease/

Parkinson's Organizations Worldwide

Young-Onset Parkinson's Organizations

American Parkinson Disease Association Young Parkinson's Information & Referral Center
Glenbrook Hospital
2100 Pfingsten Rd.
Glenview IL 60025   Phone: (800) 223-9776
E-mail: apdaypd@aol.com
Website: http://members.aol.com/apdaypd

Euroyappers Advisory Board (young-onset division of the European Parkinson's Disease Association)
Contact: Brita Nybom
EPDA
PB 905
20101 Turku
Finland   Phone: +358-2-274-0412
E-mail: Brita.nybom@Parkinson.fi

Werkgroep Yoppers (young-onset group in the Netherlands)
Parkinson Patiënten Vereniging
Postbus 46
3980 CA Bunnik
The Netherlands   Phone: 0031-30-656-13-69
Fax: 0031-30-657-13-06   E-mail: info@parkinson-vereniging.nl

From Hans van der Genugten: "The Yoppers have several regional support-group meetings and an annual national meeting for young-onset patients."

YAPP&RS—Young Alert Parkinson's Partners & Relatives
Contact: Young Onset Project Manager
c/o Parkinson's Disease Society
215 Vauxhall Bridge Rd.
London SW1V 1EJ
United Kingdom   Phone: +44 (0)207-932-1304
Website: http://youngonset-parkinsons.org.uk/

From Emma Bennion: "YAPP&Rs is the young-onset self-help group of the Parkinson's Disease Society of the UK. It is a special interest group for people with Parkinson's and their families who are of 'working age' and below."

Young Parkinson Housing Project Inc.
President: Jenny Armstrong / Vice President & contact: Chris Robie
PO Box 134
Darling
Victoria, Australia
E-mail: robespierre@optushome.com.au

This group was created by a young-Parkinson's support group in
order to find solutions to the urgent need for quality care and housing for young Parkies.

Multinational Parkinson's Organizations

European Parkinson's Disease Association (EPDA)
President: Mary Baker
215 Vauxhall Bridge Rd.
London SW1V 1EJ
United Kingdom
Phone: +44 (0)207-932-1304
Website: http://www.shef.ac.uk/misc/groups/epda/home.html

and

European Parkinson's Disease Association
c/o Parkinson Patienten Verenigung
PO Box 46
3980 CA Bunnik
Netherlands

The Nordic Parkinson Council
Website: Nordic Federation Home Page: http://www.nordiskparkinson.dk
"A council of cooperation between all Parkinson associations in the
six Nordic countries: Denmark, Sweden, Norway, Finland, Iceland,
and the Faroese Islands."

PLWP—People Living with Parkinson's
Website: http://www.plwp.org
An online organization whose aims are to: provide information to
the Parkinson's community; encourage support and friendship for
people living with Parkinson's, their partners, family, and friends;
encourage and support Parkinson's awareness; encourage and assist
fund-raising for Parkinson's research.

**We MOVE—Worldwide Education and Awareness for
Movement Disorders**
204 West 84th St.
New York NY 10024
In the United States: (800) 437-MOV2

Outside the United States: (212) 875-8312
E-mail: wemove@wemove.org Website: http://www.wemove.org

World Parkinson Disease Association
via Zuretti, 35
20125 Milano, Italy   Phone: (39) 02-66713111
E-mail: info@wpda.org   Website: http://www.wpda.org

Member directory by country: http://www.wpda.org/members.html
Note: Countries in which English is a primary language are listed first, in alphabetical order.

Australia

Parkinson's Australia Inc. (new national organization)
c/o Parkinson's New South Wales Inc.
Concord Hospital, Bld 64, Hospital Rd.,
Concord, New South Wales 2139 Phone: (02) 9767-7881
E-mail: parkinsonsnsw@bigpond.com
Website: http:// www.parkinsons.org.au

Affiliated Regional Organizations:

Parkinson's Australian Capital Territory
PO Box 717
Mawson ACT 2607   Phone: (02) 6290-1984
Website:
http://www.parkinsons.org.au/document/about_parkinsons_act.html

Parkinson's New South Wales Inc.
Concord Hospital
Bld 64, Hospital Rd.
Concord, New South Wales 2139 Phone: (02) 9767-7881
E-mail: parkinsonsnsw@aol.com
Website: http://www.parkinsonsnsw.org.au

Parkinson's Queensland
120 Main St.
Kangaroo Point
Queensland 4169   Phone: (07) 3391-38777
E-mail: pqi@parkinsons-qld.org.au
Website: http://www.parkinsons-qld.org.au/

Parkinson's South Australia
Neurological Resource Centre
23a King William Rd.
Unley SA 5061   Phone: (08) 8357-8909
E-mail: nrc@camtech.net.au
Website: http://www.span.com.au/nrc/park_intro.html

Parkinson's Tasmania
17 St Helens St.
Lindsfarne TAS 7015   Phone: (03) 6243-6510
E-mail: pdtas@netspace.net.au

Parkinson's Victoria
20 Kingston Rd.
Cheltenham VIC 3192   Phone: (03) 9551-1122
Website: http://www.parkinsons-vic.org.au/main.html

Parkinson's Association of Western Australia
ADA House
54-58 Havelock St.
PO Box 910
West Perth, WA 6872   Phone: (08) 9322-9322
E-mail: pawa@cyngus.uwa.edu.au
Website: http://www.quartec.com.au/parkinsons/

Canada

Parkinson Society Canada/Société Parkinson Canada National Office
4211 Yonge St., Suite 316
Toronto Ontario M2P 2A9   Phone: (416) 227-9700
E-mail: General.info@parkinson.ca
Website: www.Parkinson.ca

Alberta Affiliate Partners
Website: www.parkinson.ca/foundation/alberta.html

The Parkinson's Society of Alberta
Contacts: Mary Chibuk, Executive Director; Jim Haiste, President
Edmonton General, Room 3Y18
11111 Jasper Ave.
Edmonton Alberta T5K 0L4   Phone: (403) 482-8993
E-mail: psa@compusmart.ab.ca
Website: www.compusmart.ab.ca/psa

The Parkinson's Society of Southern Alberta
Contacts: Judy Axelson, Executive Director; Barry Johnson, Chairman
480D 36th Ave. SE
Calgary Alberta T2G 1W4   Phone: (403) 243-9901
E-mail: pssa@canuck.com

British Columbia Affiliate Partners
Website: www.parkinson.ca/foundation/bc.html

Victoria Epilepsy and Parkinson's Centre
Contacts: Sandra Bitz, Executive Director; Bill Pettinger, Chair
813 Darwin Ave.

Victoria BC V8X 2X7   Phone: (250) 475-6677
E-mail: sbitz@vepc.ba.ca Website: www.vepc.bc.ca

British Columbia Parkinson's Disease Association
Contacts: Lois Raphael, Executive Director; Anu Khanna, President
890 West Pender St., Suite 600
Vancouver BC V6C 1K4   Phone: (604) 662-3240
E-mail: lraphael@parkinsonsbc.com

Manitoba Chapter
Website: http://www.parkinson.ca/foundation/manitoba.html

Winnipeg Chapter
825 Sherbrook St., Suite 204
Winnipeg MB R3A 1M5   Phone: (204) 667-6247

Maritime Region
Contact: Gail Gardiner, Executive Director
Maritime Regional Office
5475 Spring Garden Rd., Suite 407
Cornwallis Building
Halifax NS B3J 3T2   Phone: (902) 422-3656
E-mail: parkinson.foundation@ns.sympatico.ca
Web page: http://www.parkinson.ca/foundation/maritimes.html

Newfoundland/Labrador Region
Website: www.parkinson.ca/foundation/newfoundland.html

Newfoundland/Labrador Regional Office
Contact: Hugh Cumming, Executive Director
PO Box 2568, Stn C
St. John's NF A1C 6K1   Phone: (709) 754-4428
E-mail: parkinson@nf.aibn.com

Ontario Regional Offices
Website: www.parkinson.ca/foundation/ontario.html

Central & Northern Ontario Region
Contact: Debbie Davis, Acting Executive Director
4211 Yonge St., Suite 316
Toronto ON M2P 2A9
Phone: (416) 227-9700   E-mail: debbie.davis@parkinson.ca

South Western Ontario Region
Contact: Carolyn Conners, Executive Director
4500 Blakie Rd., Unit #117
Meadowbrook Business Park
London ON N6L 1G5   Phone: (519) 652-9437
E-mail: parkinso@hotmail.com

Ontario Affiliate Partner
Parkinson's Society of Ottawa-Carleton
Contacts: Ken Gorman, Acting Executive Director; Grant Walsh,
President
1053 Carling Ave.
Ottawa ON K1Y 4E9   Phone: (613) 722-9238
E-mail: psoc@lri.ca or kgorman@lri.ca
Website: www.parkinsons.ca

Quebec Division Regional Office
Contact: Stephane Bordeleau, Executive Director
Fondation Canadienne du Parkinson
1253 McGill College, Suite 402
Montreal QC H3B 2Y5   Phone: (514) 861-4422
E-mail: danielle.forget@parkinson.ca
Website: www.parkinson.ca/foundation/quebec.html

Saskatchewan Affiliate Partner
Website: www.parkinson.ca/foundation/sask.html

Saskatchewan Parkinson's Disease Foundation
Contacts: Dr. David Russell, President; Dr. Ali Rajput, Secretary-
Treasurer:Ruth McGowan
Box 102, 103 Hospital Dr.
Saskatoon SK S7N 0W8   Phone: (306) 966-8160

Ireland

Parkinson's Association of Ireland
Carmichael Center
North Brunswich St.
Dublin 7   Phone: (353) 01-872-2234
Website: http://www.officeobjects.com/PARKINSONS/

Jamaica

Parkinson's Society of Jamaica
7 Glendon Circle Hope Pastures
Kingston 6

New Zealand

The Parkinsonism Society of New Zealand, Inc.
Wellington Division
PO Box 7061
Wellington South
Website: http://webnz.com/parkinsons/

South Africa

Parkinson Association South Africa
Private Bag X36
Bryanston 2021   Phone: 27 (011) 787-8792
E-mail: parkins@global.co.za
Website: www.parkinsons.co.za/Default.htm

United Kingdom

Parkinson's Disease Society of the United Kingdom (PDS)
PDS National Office
215 Vauxhall Bridge Rd.
London SW1V 1EJ
Phone: 020-7931-8080; helpline (toll-free in UK): 0808-800-0303
(Monday–Friday 9:30 A.M.–5:30 P.M.)
E-mail: enquiries@parkinsons.org.uk
For details of local officer and/or branch, e-mail:
branch.info@parkinsons.org.uk
Website: http://www.parkinsons.org.uk/

United States

American Parkinson Disease Association (APDA)
1250 Hylan Blvd.
Staten Island NY 10305
Phone: (718) 981-8001; toll-free: (800) 223-APDA (2732)
Website: http://www.apdaparkinson.com

Michael J. Fox Foundation for Parkinson's Research
Chelsea Piers, Pier 62, Suite 305
New York NY 10011   Phone: (212) 604-9182
and
1001 Pennsylvania Ave., NW
Washington DC 20004   Phone: (202) 628-2079
Website: http://www.michaeljfox.org/

National Parkinson Foundation (NPF)
1501 NW Ninth Ave.
Bob Hope Rd.
Miami FL 33136
Phone: (305) 547-6666; toll-free: (800) 327-4545
Website: http://www.parkinson.org

The Parkinson Alliance
211 College Rd. East
Princeton NJ 08540   Phone: (800) 579-8440
Website: http://www.parkinsonalliance.net/html/home.html

Parkinson's Action Network (PAN)
300 North Lee St., Suite 500
Alexandria VA 22314   Phone: (800) 850-4726
E-mail: info@parkinsonsaction.org
Website: http://www.parkinsonsaction.org

Parkinson's Disease Foundation (PDF)
710 West 168th St.
New York NY 10032-9982   Phone: (212) 923-4700
E-mail: info@pdf.org   Website: http://www.pdf.org/

PDF—Midwest office
833 West Washington Blvd.
Chicago IL 60607

The Parkinson's Institute
1170 Morse Ave.
Sunnyvale CA 94089-1605   Phone: (408) 734-2800
Website: http://www.parkinsonsinstitute.org/

Parkinson's Unity Walk
30 West 90 St.
New York NY 10024   Phone: (212) 580-6505
E-mail: mzobel@aol.com
Website: http://www.parkinsonwalk.org

Argentina
Groupo Autoayuda Parkinson Argentina
Fundacion Thompson
La Rioja 951
1221 Buenos Aires   Phone: ++541-956-0120

Grupo "Vivencias" Para Enfermos de Parkinson
Arroyo 980 4a Piso
1007 Buenos Aires   Phone: (+54) 11-4393-9422
E-mail: sidovi@fibertel.com.ar Website: http://www.datasalud.com.ar

Austria
Austrian Parkinson Patients Association
Marzstrasse 49
A-1150 Wein

Parkinson Selbsthilfe Strreich
Att: Hannes B Zeggl
Innrain 43
A-6020 Innsbruck   Phone: (+43) 512-579464
E-mail: zeggl@parkinson-sh.at or zeggl@t-online.at

Belgium

Association Parkinson Belge
Avenue Jan Stobbaertslaan 43
B-1030 Brussels   Phone: 02-245-59-45

Belgische Parkinson Vereniging (Flemish Community)
Zeedijk 286
8400 Ostend   Phone: (32) 59-70-51-81

Association Parkinson Belge
Rue Champs des Alouettes 70A
B-4557 Fraiture   Phone: 085-51-91-11

Brazil

Associação Brasil Parkinson
Avenida Bosque da Saude
1.155 04142-092
São Paulo (Brasile)   Phone: (55) 11-578-8177
E-mail: asparkin@netway.com.br
Website: http://www.parkinson.org.br

Bulgaria

Bulgaria Fondazia Parkinsonism
Blvd. Tzarigradsko Schousse - IV km
BD-1113 Sofia   Phone: (359) 2-72-7598

Chile

Liga chilena el mal del Parkinson
Arturo Prat 1341
Santiago de Chile
Chile Sudamerica   Phone: 56-2-5557716
E-mail: pchana1@ibm.net

Colombia

Asocicion Colobiana de la Enfermedad de Parkinson
Calle 106 #31 - 45
Santefe de Bogota

Croatia

Mr. Guido Klun
P. Preradovie 34
Pula, Croatia

Czech Republic

Parkinson's Disease Society
Ruska 69
10 000 Prague 10
Czech Republic   Phone: (42) 2-75-1991

Cyprus

Cyprus Parkinson Disease Association
Attn: Mr. Marios Tannousis (coordinator)
PO Box 27653
Nicosia, Cyprus   Phone: (357) 33-71-423
E-mail: lawyiann@spidernet.com.cy

Denmark

Dansk Parkinsoonforening
Hornemansgade 36 St
2100 Kobenhavn o   Phone: (45) 39-27-15-55
E-mail: dansk@Parkinson.dk Website: www.parkinson.dk/
Nordic Federation Home Page: www.nordiskparkinson.dk

Estonia

Estonian Parkinson's Society
Sole 15-1
Tallinn EE0006   Phone: (3722) 49-15-03

Finland

Suomen Parkinson-Liitto Ry
Contact: Brita Nybom
Erityisosaamiskeskus Suvituuli
PL 905
FIN-20101 TURKU   Phone: 358-2-274-0400
E-mail: parkinson-liitto@parkinson.fi
Website: www.parkinson.fi
Nordic Federation Home Page: www.nordiskparkinson.dk

France

France Parkinson
37 Bis, Rue la Fontaine
75016 Paris   Phone: (33) 1-45-20-22-20
E-mail: france-parkinson@manador.fr

Germany

Deutche Parkinson Vereiningung
Moselstrasse 31
41464 Neuss   Phone: (49) 2131-4-10-16

Hong Kong

The Parkinson's Disease Society of Hong Kong
703 East Town Building
41 Lockhart Rd.
Wanchai

Hungary

Hungarian Parkinson Disease Society
Balassa J.U. 6
Budapest
E-mail: annam@neur.sote.hu

Iceland

The Parkinson Association in Iceland
PO Box 10182
130 Reykjavik   Phone: (354) 55-24-440
Nordic Federation Home Page: www.nordiskparkinson.dk

India

Parkinson's Disease Foundation of India
Jaslok Hospital and Research Center, 12th Floor
Peddar Rd. (Bulbhai Desai)
Bombay Maharashtra 400 026   Phone: (91) 22-4963333
Website: http://indobuzz.com/pdfi/main.htm

P.K. Kanodia awak
Lion's Club, Dist. 322 E
Lai Bazar, PO
Bettiah, Bihar

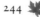

Israel

Israel Parkinson Group
PO Box 635
Kiriat Bialik 27100   Phone: (972) 2-53-35-274
E-mail: ido81@netvision.net.il

Italy

Associazione Italiana Parkinsoniani
Via Zuretti 35
20125 Milan   Phone: (39) 02-6671-3111
E-mail: aip@planet.it   Website: www.parkinson.it/aip/

Associazione Azione Parkinson
Via Sesto Celere 6
00152 Roma

Unione Parkinsoniani
Via Aueelio Saffi 43
43100 Parma

Japan

Japan Parkinson's Association
Satoshi Fujii
979-227 Misawa, Hino-Shi
Tokyo 191
E-mail: jpda@mud.biglobe.ne.jp
Website: www2.osk.3web.ne.jp/~parkin97/mypage.index_e.html

Luxembourg

Association Luxembourgeoise de la Maladie de Parkinson
42 Rue de Soleil
7250 Walferbange

Association Luxembourgeoise de la Maladie de Parkinson
BP 1348
L-1013 Luxembourg   Phone: (352) 54-62-21

Mexico

Numa Usi
Paseo de la Soladad - 86
la Herradura 53020
E-mail: ampac@data.net.mx
Website: www.ampacparkinson.org.mx

The Netherlands

Parkinson Patiënten Vereniging
Kosterijland 12 D
Postbus 46
3980 CA Bunnik   Phone: (31) 030-6561369

Norway

Norges Parkinsonforbund
Schweigaardsgt. 34
Bygg F, Oppg 1
0191 OSLO   Phone: (47) 2-217-5861
Nordic Federation Home Page: www.nordiskparkinson.dk

Pakistan

Pakistan PD Association
c/o Department of Neurology
Jinnah Postgraduate Medical Center
Karachi-35, Pakistan
E-mail: nrpwf@inet.com.pk

Peru

Asociacion Peruana Para la Enfermedad de Parkinson
Dr. Carlos Cosentino
Rousseau 488 - San Borja
Lima

Poland

Regional Parkinson's Disease Patients Association in Warsaw
Jodkowa 22/1
02-907 Warsaw   Phone: (48) 22-22-42-1331

Cracow Parkinson's Disease Association
Dr Anna Krygowska-Wajs
Klinika Neurologii
ul. Botaniczna 3
31-503 Krakow   Phone: (48) 12-61-88687

Portugal

Associação Portuguesa de Doentes de Parkinson
R. Duarte Galvao 34-7 Dto
1500 Lisbon   Phone: (351) 21-7578617

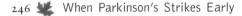

Russia

Division of Movement Disorders of the Russian Society
of Neurologists
Lininsky 8
Moscow   Phone: (7) 095-237-2730

Singapore

Parkinson's Disease Society
13/15 Kung Chong Rd.
Singapore 159149   Phone: (65) 47-98-611

Slovenia

Parkinson's Disease Society of Slovenia
Institute of Clinical Neurophysiology
61105 Ljublijana   Phone: (386) 61-316152

Spain

Parkinson Espana
Cl de al Torre 14
08006 Barcelona

Asociacion Parkinson Madrid
Estrecho de Gibraltar, 21-18
28027 Madrid   Phone: (34) 1-336-8384

Sweden

Svenska Parkinsonforbundet (Swedish Parkinson Foundation)
Nybrokajen 7, 3 trp
S-111 48 Stockholm   Phone: (46) 611-93-31
E-mail: parkinsons@communique.se
Website: http://www.parkinsonforbundt.se
Nordic Federation Home Page: www.nordiskparkinson.dk

Switzerland

Association Suisse de la Maladie de Parkinson
Case Postale
8128 Hinteregg   Phone: 01-9840169

Schweizerische Parkinsonvereinigung
Gewerbestrasse 12a
PO Box 123
CH-8132 Egg   Phone: (41) 1-984-0169
E-mail: info@parkinson.ch   Website: www.parkinson.ch

Taiwan

Taiwan Parkinson's Association
Department of Neurology
National Taiwan University Hospital
No. 7, Chung-Shan South Rd.
Taipei 100, Taiwan, R.O.C.   Phone: (886) 2-239-70-800 ext. 5337
E-mail: rmwu@ha.mc.ntu.edu.tw

Turkey

Parkinson's Disease Society
c/o Bilim Sok Doost Apt No.8 D.8
Erenköy
81070 Istanbul   Phone: (90) 212-588-3770

Ukraine

The Association for Parkinsonian Disabled
67 Vyshgorodskaya str.
254114 Kiev   Phone: (38044) 430-40-68

Yugoslavia

Serbian Association Against Parkinson's Disease
Institute of Neurology
Dr Subotica St. 6
11000 Beograd   Phone: (381) 11-68-55-54

Note: Directory information for many of these organizations was located on the following websites:

World Parkinson's Disease Association (WPDA) website:
http://www.wpda.org/members.html

European Parkinson's Disease Association (EPDA) website:
http://www.shef.ac.uk/misc/groups/epda/home.html

Awakenings website—patients' groups:
http://www.parkinsonsdisease.com

Endnotes

Introduction

1. Cousins, Norman. *Head First: The Biology of Hope.* New York: Dutton, 1989, p. 12.
2. U.S. National Institutes of Health. National Institute of Neurological Disorders and Stroke. *Parkinson's Disease: A Research Planning Workshop, August 28–30, 1995.* Retrieved online: <http://www.ninds.nih.gov/health_and_medical/pubs/parkinson_w orkshop_proceeding.htm> (12 February 2001).
3. Greene, Dennis. "I Didn't Come Here for This." In *Voices from the Parking Lot,* edited by Dennis Greene, et al. Princeton, NJ: The Parkinson's Alliance, 2000, 4.

Chapter 1

1. van der Werf, Martin. "Arizona Losing a Legend." *Arizona Republic* (Phoenix), 1991. Reprinted in *Addresses and Special Orders Presented in Honor of the Honorable Morris "Mo" K. Udall.* One Hundred Second Congress, U.S. Government Printing Office, 1993, 245.
2. Martone, Nancy. "How to Recognize a Person With Parkinson's." (Speech to Humble, Texas, Intercontinental Rotary), 13 April 1994. Retrieved online: PARKINSN Archive <http://parkinsn.coles.org.uk/> (12 December 1999).
3. From the following sources: World Health Organization. "Press release: Parkinson's Disease—a Unique Survey." WHO Website <http://www.who.ch/> (26 September 2000); "Description of Parkinson's." Parkinson's Foundation website. Retrieved online: <http://www.parkinson.ca/pd/parkinson.html> (3 March 2001); "The National Parkinson Foundation States Parkinson's Disease Becoming More Prevalent Among the 'Young.'" *PRNewswire,* 28 November 1998. Retrieved online: PARKINSN Archive <http://parkinsn.coles.org.uk/> (2 December 1998).

4. Smith, Carol. "Parkinson's Disease: The Silent Epidemic." *Seattle Post-Intelligencer Reporter*, 1 April 1999. Retrieved online: PARKINSN Archive <http://parkinsn.coles.org.uk/> (12 April 1999).

5. YAPP&RS: Young Alert Parkinson's Partners & Relatives Homepage. <http://james.parkinsons.org.uk/PDSUK/pdsyappers.htm> (25 February 2001).

6. Boots, David. "Me and My Banjo." *Movers and Shakers Newsletter.* December 1994. Posted to PIEN, 3 October 1996. Retrieved online: *PARKINSN Archive.* <http://parkinsn.coles.org.uk/> (7 December 1998).

7. Pikunis, Richard. Testimony. U.S. Congress. Senate Appropriations Committee, Labor, Health and Human Services Subcommittee. "Hearing on Stem Cell Research: Patenting and Health Implications." (12 January 1999). Text from: *Federal Document Clearing House Political Transcripts.* Retrieved online: CIS Congressional Universe <http://web.lexis-nexis.com> (8 March 2001).

8. Ashworth, Blair. "I Thought I was Far Too Young for Parkinson's." *The Daily Mail* (London, England), 1 December 1998. Retrieved online: <http://freespace.virgin.net/dennis.ogden/parkinsons/> (5 January 1999).

9. Gilman, Sid, et al. "Diagnostic Criteria for Parkinson's Disease." *Archives of Neurology* 56 (1999): 33–39. Retrieved online: Archives of Neurology website. <http://archneur.ama-assn.org/> (18 February 2001).

10. Bennion, Emma. "Young Onset Parkinson's Disease." Awakenings website. Retrieved online: <http://www.parkinsonsdisease.com> (20 November 1999).

11. Boots, "Me and My Banjo."

12. Ashworth, "I Thought."

13. Pikunis, "Testimony."

14. Ashworth, "I Thought."

15. Bennion, Emma. "Attitude in PD—A Personal Perspective." Awakenings website. Retrieved online: <http://www.parkinsonsdisease.com> (20 November 1999).

16. Martone, Nancy. "How to Recognize."

17. Tompkins, Phil. "Advice To The Newly Diagnosed." PD Index: A Directory of Parkinson's Disease Information on the Internet. Retrieved online: <http://www.pdindex.com> (27 October 2000).

Chapter 2

1. Martone, Nancy. "How to Recognize a Person With Parkinson's." (Speech to Humble, Texas, Intercontinental Rotary), 13 April 1994. Retrieved online: PARKINSN Archive <http://parkinsn.coles.org.uk/> (12 December 1999).

2. Udall, Anne. "A Daughter's Fond Memories." *Arizona Law Record.* Reprinted in: *Addresses and Special Orders Presented in Honor of the Honorable Morris "Mo" K. Udall.* One Hundred Second Congress, U.S. Government Printing Office, 1993, 168.

3. Ashworth, Blair. "I Thought I was Far Too Young for Parkinson's." *The Daily Mail* (London, England), 1 December 1998. Retrieved online: <http://freespace.virgin.net/dennis.ogden/parkinsons/> (5 January 1999).

4. Martone, Nancy. "How to Recognize."

5. Cordy, Jim. Testimony. U.S. Congress. House Appropriations Committee. Labor, Health and Human Services Subcommittee "Hearing on FY99 Labor, Health and Human Services Appropriations" (4 February 1998) Retrieved online: Parkinson's Action Network website <http://www.parkinsonsaction.org> (19 November 2000).

6. Houston, Stan. "Parkinson's Can Turn Life Topsy-Turvy." *Houston Chronicle.* 17 November 1996. Retrieved online: PARKINSN Archive. <http://parkinsn.coles.org.uk/> (9 April 1999).

7. Martone, Nancy. "How to Recognize."

8. Pikunis, Richard. "Testimony."

9. Martone, Nancy. "How to Recognize."

10. "European Study Shows Extent of Problems Faced by PWP." *The PDF News,* Fall/Winter 1998–99, 10.

11. Martone, Nancy. "How to Recognize."

12. Kondracke, Morton. "Cruel and Unusual." *The Washingtonian,* April 1996, 75.

13. Kondracke. "Cruel and Unusual." 76.

14. Jones, Celia. "Parkinson's Progressive?" (unpublished essay).

15. Kondracke. "Cruel and Unusual." 76.

16. Houston. "Parkinson's Can Turn."

Chapter 3

1. Fox, Michael J. Testimony. U.S. Congress. Senate Appropriations Committee, Subcommittee on Labor, Health and Human Services, Education and Related Agencies. "Hearing on Parkinson's Disease Research and Treatment" (28 September 1999). Text from: *Federal Document Clearing House Political Transcripts*. Retrieved online: CIS Congressional Universe <http://web.lexis-nexis.com> (8 March 2001).

2. Boots, David. "Me and My Banjo." *Movers and Shakers Newsletter*. December 1994. Posted to PIEN, 3 October 1996. Retrieved online: *PARKINSN Archive*. <http://parkinsn.coles.org.uk/> (7 December 1998).

3,4. Scheife, Richard T., et al. "Impact of Parkinson's Disease and Its Pharmacologic Treatment on Quality of Life and Economic Outcomes." *American Journal of Health Systems Pharmacology*, 57(2000): 953–962. Retrieved online: Medscape <www.medscape.com> (18 November 2000).

5. "New PDF Survey Shows That Only One in Three PWPs Sees a Parkinson's Specialist." *The PDF News*, Summer/Fall 2000, 10.

6. Ali, Lonnie. Testimony. U.S. Congress. House Appropriations Subcommittee for the Departments of Labor, Health and Human Services, Education and Related Agencies. "Hearing on the Udall Bill." 23 April 1997. Retrieved online: PARKINSN Archive, <http://parkinsn.coles.org.uk/> (18 March 2001).

7. Cohen, Perry. "Quality, Delivery and Access to Parkinson's Care." (website) <http://www.parkinsonscare.org/index.htm> (14 November 2000).

8. Broberg, Brad. "Center of Hope: The New Booth Gardner Parkinson's Care Center Is the Largest West of the Mississippi." *Puget Sound Business Journal*, August 2000. Retrieved online: PARKINSN Archive, 14 August 2000. <http://parkinsn.coles.org.uk/> (18 November 2000).

9. John Grooms Housing Authority. "Building Partnerships—With Care Agencies." Website. <http://www.johngrooms.org.uk/housing/partnership/parkinsons.htm> (14 November 2000).

10. Greene, Dennis. "A Terrible Beauty." Speech to Parkinson's Association of Western Australia. (1998).

Chapter 4

1. Rezak, Michael. "Parkinson's Disease in the Young." *APDA Young Parkinson's Newsletter,* Summer/Fall 1998. Retrieved online: APDA Young Parkinson's Information & Referral Center website. <http://www.members.aol.com/apdaypd> (15 January 2001).

2. Snyder, Joan Blessington. "Kids." In *Voices From The Parking Lot.* Edited by Dennis Greene, et. al. Princeton, NJ: The Parkinson's Alliance, 2000. 20.

3. Martone, Nancy. "How to Recognize."

4. Finch, Jerry. "Loving and Sexuality." In *Voices From The Parking Lot.* Edited by Dennis Greene, et. al. Princeton, NJ: The Parkinson's Alliance, 2000. 24.

5. Reese, Susan. "Parkinson's Disease: Issues in Caring for the Patient With Young-Onset Parkinson's Disease." *Home Healthcare Consultant Online.* Retrieved online: http://www.mmhc.com/hhcc/articles/HHCC9904/reese.html (29 November 1999).

6. Kamphuis, Ida. "Sons and Daughters." *APDA Young Parkinson's Newsletter,* Spring 1998. Retrieved online: APDA Young Parkinson's Information & Referral Center website. <http://www.members.aol.com/apdaypd> (18 November 2000).

7. Boots, David. "May I Have This Dance?" (Personal Homepage.) Retrieved online: <http://www.sonic.net/~bootst3k/dance.html> (5 November 2000).

Chapter 5

1. "Pacific Parkinson's Research Institute Commissions Study." Parkinson's Foundation of Canada Website. < http://www.parkinson.ca/pnet85/pnet85-2.html#pacific>. Summary posted to PARKINSN Archive, 8 May 1998. Retrieved online: <http://parkinsn.coles.org.uk/> (25 November 2000).

2. Smith, Carol. "Parkinson's disease: The silent epidemic."

3. Montgomery, Erwin B. "The Young Parkinson's Patient." *Parkinson News & Views,* Newsletter of the Southern Arizona Chapter APDA, June/July 1994. Retrieved online: PARKINSN Archive <http://parkinsn.coles.org.uk/> (12 December 1999).

4. Samuelson, Joan. Testimony. U.S. Congress. House Appropriations Committee. Labor, Health and Human Services Subcommittee "Hearing on FY99 Labor, Health and Human Services Appropriations" (4 February 1998). Retrieved online: Parkin-

son's Action Network website
<http://www.parkinsonsaction.org> (19 November 2000).

5. "Parkinson's Disease: The Need For a Fair, Adequate Research Budget." Parkinson's Action Network website. Retrieved online: <http://www.pansonic.org> (26 November 1999).

6. Samuelson, Joan. Interview by Daniel Zwerdling, *All Things Considered*, National Public Radio, 12 January 1997. Transcript retrieved online: Parkinson's Action Network website <http://www.pansonic.org> (3 November 1999).

7. Fox, Michael J. Testimony. U.S. Congress, 1999.

8. "Ali Receives Medal." *AOL 1996 Olympics Report*. 4 August 1996. Retrieved online PARKINSN Archive <http://parkinsn.coles.org.uk/> (23 November 2000).

9. "Ali Receives Medal."

10. Gillis, Charlie. "Celebrity spokesmen can raise the funds that allow doctors to continue vital research—Public, governments tend to listen when the speaker is a star." *National Post*, 27 November 1998. Retrieved online. PARKINSN Archive <http://parkinsn.coles.org.uk/> (7 December 1998).

11. "Ali Honored For Disease Fight." *Associated Press Newswire*. 24 September 1996. Retrieved online: PARKINSN Archive <http://parkinsn.coles.org.uk/> (29 September 1996).

12. Boots, David. "The Wish." Personal Homepage. Retrieved online: <http://www.sonic.net/~bootst3k/thewish.html> (5 November 2000).

Chapter 6

1. Blake-Krebs, Barbara. "PD on the Internet: A World-Wide Support Group." *Parkinson's Update: Newsletter of Parkinson's Association of Greater Kansas City*, Fall 1996.

2. Ashworth, Blair. "I Thought I was Far Too Young for Parkinson's." *The Daily Mail* (London, England), 1 December 1998. Retrieved online: <http://freespace.virgin.net/dennis.ogden/parkinsons/> (5 January 1999).

3. Bennion, Emma. "Young Onset Parkinson's Disease." Awakenings website. Retrieved online: <http://www.parkinsonsdisease.com> (20 November 1999).

4. Kondracke, Morton. "Cruel and Unusual." *The Washingtonian*, April 1996, 75.

5. Dolezal, Bob. "Guest Comment: Parkinson's Bill is Critical to Advance Research." *Arizona Daily Star*, 14 July 1996, D3.

6. U.S. National Institutes of Health. National Institute of Neurological Disorders and Stroke. Parkinson's Disease Research
   Agenda, 2000–2005. March 2000. Retrieved online.
   <http://www.ninds.nih.gov/whatsnew/pdagenda2000/nihparkin-
   sonsagenda.htm> (23 November 2000).
7. Fox, Michael J. Testimony, U.S. Congress, 1999.

Chapter 7

1. Schrag, Annette, et. al. "Young Parkinson's Disease Revisited—
   Clinical Features, Natural History and Mortality." *Movement
   Disorders* 13(1998), 885.
2. Langston, William. Testimony. U.S. Congress. Senate Appropriations Committee, Subcommittee on Labor, Health and Human
   Services, Education and Related Agencies. "Hearing on Parkinson's Disease Research and Treatment" (28 September 1999).
   Text from: *Federal Document Clearing House Political Transcripts*. Retrieved online: CIS Congressional Universe
   <http://web.lexis-nexis.com> (8 March 2001).
3. Koller, William C. "Surgical Treatments for Parkinson's Disease." *NPF Parkinson Report*, Winter 2000, 8.
4. Ross, Jane. "My DBS Surgery" (Webpage). Last updated 30
   November 2000. Retrieved online:
   <http://www.geocities.com/SoHo/Village/6263/pienet/ross/index.ht
   ml> (1 April 2001).
5. Langston. Testimony. U.S. Congress, 1999.
6. Freed, Curt R., et al. "Transplantation of Embryonic Dopamine
   Neurons for Severe Parkinson's Disease." *The New England
   Journal of Medicine* 344 (2001): 710–719. Retrieved online:
   Journals@Ovid Fulltext <http://gateway1.ovid.com:80/ovidweb.cgi>
   (1 April 2001).
7, 8. Coles, Joanna. "We'd do it again." *The Times (London).* 15
   March 2001. Retrieved online: LEXIS/NEXIS Academic Universe. <http://web.lexis-nexis.com/universe> (3 April 2001).

Chapter 8

1. Boots, David. "A Voice in the Park…A Piece of Cloth." Personal
   Homepage. Retrieved online:
   <http://www.sonic.net/~bootst3k/cloth.html> (5 November 2000)
2. Fox, Michael J. Testimony. U.S. Congress, 1999.
3. Fischbach, Gerald. Testimony. U.S. Congress. Senate Appropria-

tions Committee, Subcommittee on Labor, Health and Human Services, Education and Related Agencies. "Hearing on Parkinson's Disease Research and Treatment." (28 September 1999). Text from: *Federal Document Clearing House Political Transcripts*. Retrieved online: CIS Congressional Universe <http://web.lexis-nexis.com> (8 March 2001).

4. From the following sources: World Health Organization. "Press release: Parkinson's Disease—a Unique Survey." WHO Website <http://www.who.ch/> (26 September 2000); "Description of Parkinson's." Parkinson's Foundation website. Retrieved online: <http://www.parkinson.ca/pd/parkinson.html> (3 March 2001); "The National Parkinson Foundation States Parkinson's Disease Becoming More Prevalent Among the 'Young.'" *PRNewswire*, 28 November 1998. Retrieved online: PARKINSN Archive <http://parkinsn.coles.org.uk/> (2 December 1998).

5. Osterweil, Neil. "Researchers Find Large Piece of the Gulf War Syndrome Puzzle: Vets' Brain Changes May Lead to Parkinson's Disease Down the Road." *WebMD Medical News*, 24 September 2000. Retrieved online: WebMD <http://my.webmd.com> (30 September 2000).

6. Langston, William. Testimony. U.S. Congress, 1999.

7. Langston, William. "Research and Hope for All of Us." (Speech at Parkinson's Unity Walk, New York City, 1997.) Retrieved online: PARKINSN Archive <http://parkinsn.coles.org.uk/> (9 April 1999).

8. "Gene Therapy Could Give Hope to Parkinson's Patients." Canadian Broadcasting Corporation website, 26 October 2000. Retrieved online: <http://cbc.ca/> (27 October 2000).

9. Ricer, Paul. "Parkinson's Disease: Possible 'Cure' in Political Arena." *The Atlanta Journal-Constitution*, 18 February, 2001. Retrieved online: PARKINSN Archive. <http://parkinsn.coles.org.uk/> (18 February 2001).

10. U.S. National Institutes of Health. "NIH Fact Sheet on Human Pluripotent Stem Cell Research Guidelines." 23 August 2000. Retrieved online. <http://www.nih.gov/news/stemcell/stemfactsheet.htm> (30 August 2000).

References

"Ali Honored For Disease Fight." *Associated Press Newswire.* 24
September 1996. Retrieved online: PARKINSN Archive,
<http://parkinsn.coles.org.uk/> (23 November 2000).

"Ali Receives Medal." *AOL 1996 Olympics Report.* 4 August
1996. Retrieved online: PARKINSN Archive,
<http://parkinsn.coles.org.uk/> (23 November 2000).

Ali, Lonnie. Testimony. U.S. Congress. House Appropriations Subcommittee for the Departments of Labor, Health & Human Services, Education and Related Agencies. "Hearing on the Udall
Bill." 23 April 1997. Retrieved online: PARKINSN Archive,
<http://parkinsn.coles.org.uk/> (18 March 2001).

Ashworth, Blair. "I Thought I Was Far Too Young for Parkinson's."
The Daily Mail (London, England), 1 December 1998.
Retrieved online: <http://freespace.virgin.net/dennis.ogden/parkin-
sons/> (5 January 1999).

Bennion, Emma. "Attitude in PD—a Personal Perspective." Awakenings website. Retrieved online:
<http://www.parkinsonsdisease.com> (20 November 1999).

———."Young Onset Parkinson's Disease." Awakenings website.
Retrieved online: <http://www.parkinsonsdisease.com> (20
November 1999).

Blake-Krebs, Barbara. "PD on the Internet: A World-Wide Support
Group." *Parkinson Update: Newsletter of Parkinson's Association of Greater Kansas City,* Fall 1996.

———. "PD Advocates." *Parkinson Update: Newsletter of Parkinson's Association of Greater Kansas City,* Winter 2000.

Boots, David. "May I Have This Dance?" Personal Homepage.
Retrieved online: <http://www.sonic.net/~bootst3k/dance.html>
(5 November 2000)

———."Me and My Banjo." *Movers and Shakers Newsletter,*
December 1994. Posted to PIEN, 3 October 1996. Retrieved
online: PARKINSN Archive, <http://parkinsn.coles.org.uk/> (7
December 1998).

———. "A Voice in the Park...A Piece of Cloth." Personal Home-

page. Retrieved online: <http://www.sonic.net/~bootst3k/cloth
.html> (5 November 2000).

———. "The Wish." Personal Homepage. Retrieved
online:<http://www.sonic.net/~bootst3k/thewish.html>(5 November 2000)

Broberg, Brad. "Center of Hope: The New Booth Gardner Parkinson's Care Center is the Largest West of the Mississippi." *Puget Sound Business Journal,* August 2000. Retrieved online: PARKINSN Archive, 14 August 2000. <http://parkinsn.coles.org.uk/> (18 November 2000).

Cohen, Perry. Quality, Delivery and Access to Parkinson's Care (website) <http://www.parkinsonscare.org> (14 November 2000).

Coles, Joanna. "We'd do it again." *The Times (London).* 15 March 2001. Retrieved online: *LEXIS/NEXIS Academic Universe.* <http://web.lexis-nexis.com/universe> (3 April 2001).

Cousins, Norman. *Head First: The Biology of Hope.* New York: E. P. Dutton, 1989.

"Description of Parkinson's." Parkinson's Foundation of Canada website. Retrieved online <http://www.parkinson.ca/pd/parkinson.html> (3 March 2001)

Dolezal, Bob. "Guest Comment: Parkinson's Bill is Critical to Advance Research." *Arizona Daily Star,* 14 July 1996, D3.

"European Study Shows Extent of Problems Faced by PWP." *The PDF News,* Fall/Winter 1998–99, 10+.

Finch, Jerry. "Loving and Sexuality." In *Voices From The Parking Lot,* edited by Dennis Greene, et al. Princeton, NJ: The Parkinson's Alliance, 2000. 24–27.

Freed, Curt R., et al. "Transplantation of Embryonic Dopamine Neurons for Severe Parkinson's Disease." *The New England Journal of Medicine* 344 (2001): 710–719. Retrieved online: Journals@Ovid Fulltext <http://gateway1.ovid.com:80/ovidweb.cgi> (1 April 2001)

"Gene Therapy Could Give Hope to Parkinson's Patients." Canadian Broadcasting Corporation Website, 26 October 2000. Retrieved online: <http://cbc.ca/> (27 October 2000).

Gillis, Charlie. "Celebrity Spokesmen Can Raise the Funds That Allow Doctors to Continue Vital Research." *National Post,* 27 November 1998. Retrieved online: PARKINSN Archive <http://parkinsn.coles.org.uk/> (7 December 1998).

Gilman, Sid, et al. "Diagnostic Criteria for Parkinson's Disease." *Archives of Neurology* 56 (1999): 33–39. Retrieved online: Archives of Neurology website. <http://archneur.ama-assn.org/> (18 February 2001).

Greene, Dennis. "A Terrible Beauty." Speech to Parkinson's Association of Western Australia. (1998).

———. "I Didn't Come Here For This." In *Voices From The Parking Lot,* edited by Dennis Greene, et al. Princeton, NJ: The Parkinson's Alliance, 2000. 4.

Houston, Stan. "Parkinson's Can Turn Life Topsy-Turvy." *Houston Chronicle.* 17 November 1996. Retrieved online: PARKINSN Archive. <http://parkinsn.coles.org.uk/> (9 April 1999).

———. John Grooms Housing Authority. "Building Partnerships— With Care Agencies." Website <http://www.johngrooms.org.uk/housing/partnership/parkinsons.htm> (14 November 2000).

Jones, Celia. "Parkinson's Progressive?" (unpublished essay).

Kamphuis, Ida. "Sons and Daughters." *APDA Young Parkinson's Newsletter,* Spring 1998. Retrieved online: APDA Young Parkinson's Information & Referral Center website. <http://www.members.aol.com/apdaypd> (18 November 2000).

Koller, William C. "Surgical Treatments for Parkinson's Disease." *NPF Parkinson Report.* Winter 2000, 6–9.

Koller, William C., and Montgomery, E. B. "Issues in the Early Diagnosis of Parkinson's Disease." *Neurology* 49, Suppl 1 (1997): S10–25.

Kondracke, Morton. "Cruel and Unusual." *The Washingtonian,* April 1996, 74–8.

Langston, William. "Research and Hope for All of Us." (Speech at Parkinson's Unity Walk, New York City, 1997.) Retrieved online: PARKINSN Archive <http://parkinsn.coles.org.uk/> (9 April 1999).

Lieberman, Abraham. "What is Parkinson's Disease?" In: *Young Parkinson's Handbook.* New York: The American Parkinson Disease Association, 1995, 1–9.

Martone, Nancy. "How to Recognize a Person With Parkinson's." (Speech to Humble, Texas, Intercontinental Rotary, 13 April 1994.) Retrieved online: PARKINSN Archive <http://parkinsn.coles.org.uk/> (12 December 1999).

Montgomery, Erwin B. "The Young Parkinson's Patient." *Parkinson News & Views: Newsletter of the Southern Arizona Chapter APDA,* June/July 1994. Retrieved online: PARKINSN Archive <http://parkinsn.coles.org.uk/> (12 December 1999).

"The National Parkinson Foundation States Parkinson's Disease Becoming More Prevalent Among the 'Young.'" *PRNewswire,* 28 November 1998. Retrieved online: PARKINSN Archive. <http://parkinsn.coles.org.uk/> (2 December, 1998).

"New PDF Survey Shows That Only One in Three PWPs Sees a Parkinson's Specialist." *The PDF News,* Summer/Fall 2000, p.10.

Olanow, C. Warren, and William C. Koller. "Management of Parkinson's Disease." *Neurology* 50, Suppl. 3, (March 1998).

Osterweil, Neil. "Researchers Find Large Piece of the Gulf War Syndrome Puzzle: Vets' Brain Changes May Lead to Parkinson's Disease Down the Road." *WebMD Medical News,* 24 September 2000. Retrieved online: WebMD <http://my.webmd.com> (30 September 2000).

"Pacific Parkinson's Research Institute Commissions Study." Parkinson's Foundation of Canada website. <http://www.parkinson.ca/pnet85/pnet85-2.html#pacific>. Summary posted to PARKINSN Archive, 8 May 1998. Retrieved online: <http://parkinsn.coles.org.uk/> (25 November 2000).

"Parkinson's Disease: The Need For a Fair, Adequate Research Budget." Parkinson's Action Network website. Retrieved online: <http://www.pansonic.org> (26 November 1999).

Pikunis, Richard. Testimony. U.S. Congress. Senate Appropriations Committee, Labor, Health and Human Services Subcommittee. "Hearing on Stem Cell Research: Patenting and Health Implications." (12 January 1999). Text from: *Federal Document Clearing House Political Transcripts.* Retrieved online: *CIS Congressional Universe* <http://web.lexis-nexis.com> (8 March 2001).

Reese, Susan. "Parkinson's Disease: Issues in Caring for the Patient With Young-Onset Parkinson's Disease." Retrieved online: *Home Healthcare Consultant Online,* April 1999. <http://www.mmhc.com/hhcc/articles/HHCC9904/reese.html> (29 November 1999).

Rezak, Michael. "Parkinson's Disease in the Young." *APDA Young Parkinson's Newsletter,* Summer/Fall 1998. Retrieved online: APDA Young Parkinson's Information & Referral Center website. <http://www.members.aol.com/apdaypd> (15 January 2001).

Ricer, Paul. "Parkinson's Disease: Possible 'Cure' in Political Arena." *The Atlanta Journal-Constitution,* 18 February 2001. Retrieved online: PARKINSN Archive. <http://parkinsn.coles.org.uk/> (18 February 2001).

Ross, Jane. "My DBS Surgery." Personal webpage. Last updated 30 November 2000. Retrieved online: http://www.geocities.com/SoHo/Village/6263/pienet/ross/index.ht ml> (1 April 2001).

Samuelson, Joan. Testimony. U.S. Congress. Hearing of the U.S. Senate Special Committee on Aging and the Committee on Appropriations. "Investing in Medical Research: Saving Health Care and Human Costs." (26 September 1996). Washington D.C.: GPO, 1996, 19–34.

————. Testimony. U.S. Congress. House Appropriations Committee, Labor Health and Human Services Subcommittee. "Hearing on FY98 Appropriations." (24 April 1997) Text from: *Federal Document Clearing House Political Transcripts.* Retrieved online: CIS Congressional Universe <http://web.lexis-nexis.com> (8 March 2001).

————. Interview by Daniel Zwerdling, *All Things Considered,* National Public Radio, 12 January 1997. Transcript retrieved online: Parkinson's Action Network website <http://www.pansonic.org> (3 November 1999).

Schneider, Karen S., and Todd Gold. "Michael J. Fox Faces an Uncharted Future With Courage and Compassion As He Confronts a Cruel Foe: Parkinson's Disease." *People Weekly,* 7 December 1998: 126–136.

Scheife, Richard T., et al. "Impact of Parkinson's Disease and Its Pharmacologic Treatment on Quality of Life and Economic Outcomes." *American Journal of Health Systems Pharmacology* 57(2000): 953–962. Retrieved online: Medscape <www.medscape.com> (18 November 2000).

Schrag, Annette, et. al. "Young Parkinson's Disease Revisited—Clinical Features, Natural History and Mortality." *Movement Disorders* 13(1998): 885–894.

Shulman, L. M., et. al. "Internal Tremor in Patients With Parkinson's Disease." *Movement Disorders* 11 (1996): 3–7.

Smith, Carol. "Parkinson's Disease: The Silent Epidemic." *Seattle Post-Intelligencer Reporter,* 1 April 1999. Retrieved online: PARKINSN Archive <http://parkinsn.coles.org.uk/> (12 April 1999).

Snyder, Joan Blessington. "Kids." in *Voices From The Parking Lot,* edited by Dennis Greene et. al. Princeton, NJ: The Parkinson's Alliance, 2000. 20.

Tompkins, Phil. "Advice To The Newly Diagnosed." PD Index: A Directory of Parkinson's Disease Information on the Internet (website). Retrieved online: <http://www.pdindex.com> (27 October 2000).

Udall, Anne. "A Daughter's Fond Memories." *Arizona Law Record.* Reprinted in: *Addresses and Special Orders Presented in Honor of the Honorable Morris "Mo" K. Udall.* One Hundred Second Congress, U.S. Government Printing Office, 1993, 167–170.

U.S. Congress. House Appropriations Committee. Labor, Health and Human Services Subcommittee "Hearing on FY99 Labor, Health and Human Services Appropriations" (4 February 1998). Retrieved online: Parkinson's Action Network website <http://www.parkinsonsaction.org> (19 November 2000).

U.S. Congress. Senate Appropriations Committee, Subcommittee on Labor, Health and Human Services, Education and Related Agencies. "Hearing on Parkinson's Disease Research and Treatment" (28 September 1999). Text from: *Federal Document Clearing House Political Transcripts*. Retrieved online: CIS Congressional Universe <http://web.lexis-nexis.com> (8 March 2001).

U.S. National Human Genome Research Institute. "Research News: Parkinson's Disease?" NHGRI Website <http://www.nhgri.nih.gov/NEWS/PARK/background_info.html> (2 December, 1999).

U.S. National Institutes of Health. "NIH Fact Sheet on Human Pluripotent Stem Cell Research Guidelines." 23 August 2000. Retrieved online: NIH website. <http://www.nih.gov/news/stemcell/stemfactsheet.htm> (30 August 2000).

U.S. National Institutes of Health. National Institute of Neurological Disorders and Stroke. *Parkinson's Disease: A Research Planning Workshop, August 28–30, 1995*. Retrieved online: <http://www.ninds.nih.gov/health_and_medical/pubs/parkinson_w orkshop_proceeding.htm> (12 February 2001).

U.S. National Institutes of Health. National Institute of Neurological Disorders and Stroke. *Parkinson's Disease Research Agenda, 2000–2005*. March 2000. Retrieved online: <http://www.ninds.nih.gov/whatsnew/pdagenda2000/nihparkinsonsagenda.htm> (23 November 2000).

U.S. Public Law 105-78. Departments of Labor, Health and Human Services and Education, and Related Agencies Appropriations Act, 1998. Sec. 603 Morris K. Udall Parkinson's Disease Research Act of 1997.

U.S. Social Security Administration. "*Social Security: Understanding the Benefits.*" (pamphlet), July 2000.

van der Werf, Martin. "Arizona Loosing a Legend," *Arizona Republic*, 1991. Reprinted in: *Addresses and Special Orders Presented in Honor of the Honorable Morris "Mo" K. Udall*. One Hundred Second Congress, U.S. Government Printing Office, 1993, 242–6.

Whetten-Goldstein, K., et. al. "The Burden of Parkinson's Disease on Society, Family and the Individual." *Journal of the American Geriatric Society*. 45(7), 844–9.

World Health Organization. "Press Release: Parkinson's Disease—a Unique Survey." Retrieved online: WHO website <http://www.who.ch/> (26 September 2000).

YAPP&RS: Young Alert Parkinson's Partners & Relatives Website. <http://james.parkinsons.org.uk/PDSUK/pdsyappers.htm> (25 February, 2001).

Index

GET FIT WHILE YOU SIT: Easy Workouts from Your Chair
by Charlene Torkelson

Here is a total-body workout that can be done right from your chair, anywhere. It is perfect for office workers, travelers, and those with age-related movement limitations or special conditions. This book offers three programs. The *One-Hour Chair Program* is a full-body, low-impact workout that includes light aerobics and exercises to be done with or without weights. The *5-Day Short Program* features five compact workouts for those short on time. Finally, the *Ten-Minute Miracles* is a group of easy-to-do exercises perfect for anyone on the go.

160 pages ... 212 b/w photos ... Paperback 12.95 ... Hardcover $22.95

COMPUTER AND WEB RESOURCES FOR PEOPLE WITH DISABILITIES *by* the Alliance for Technology Access

This book shows how people can use computer technology to enhance their lives. It describes conventional and assistive technologies, gives strategies for accessing Internet resources, and features charts relating access needs to software, hardware, and communication aids. Also included is a gold mine of Web resources, publications, support organizations, government programs, and technology vendors.

The third edition is updated with extensive information about the World Wide Web and its role in expanding access to resources.

384 pages ... 40 b/w photos ... 8 charts ... Third revised edition
Paperback $20.95 ... Spiral bound $27.95 ... ASCII disk $27.95

CHINESE HERBAL MEDICINE MADE EASY: Natural and Effective Remedies for Common Illnesses
by Thomas Richard Joiner

Chinese herbal medicine is an ancient system for maintaining health and prolonging life. This book demystifies the subject, with clear explanations and easy-to-read alphabetical listings of more than 750 herbal remedies for over 250 common illnesses ranging from acid reflux and AIDS to breast cancer, pain management, sexual dysfunction, and weight loss. Whether you are a newcomer to herbology or a seasoned practitioner, you will find this book a valuable addition to your health library.

448 pages ... Paperback $24.95 ... Hardcover $34.95

To order books see last page or call (800) 266-5592

ALZHEIMER'S EARLY STAGES: First Steps in Caring and Treatment *by* Daniel Kuhn, MSW

This book is for the family and friends of those recently diagnosed with Alzheimer's. The first part discusses how the disease affects the brain, known risk factors, the latest treatments, and guidelines for prevention. An important chapter presents what it is like to live with Alzheimer's.

Part Two covers changing relationships, developing new lines of communication, taking responsibility for decisions, and encouraging the patient to try to slow the progress of the disease. Kuhn recommends starting long-term planning immediately and addresses ways that caregivers should take care of themselves.

288 pages ... Paperback $14.95 ... Hardcover $24.95

ALTERNATIVE TREATMENTS FOR FIBROMYALGIA AND CHRONIC FATIGUE SYNDROME: Insights from Practitioners and Patients *by* Mari Skelly and Andrea Helm; Foreword by Paul Brown, M.D., Ph.D.

Many people suffering from fibromyalgia and CFS are unable to find effective treatment and relief. This book combines interviews with practitioners of alternative therapies—including acupuncture, massage therapy, chiropractic, psychotherapy, and energetic healing—with personal stories from patients. These offer a firsthand look at symptoms, treatments, struggles and successes, lifestyle adaptations and medicine, diet, and activity regimens that might help others. There are also sections on obtaining health insurance and Social Security disability.

288 pages ... Paperback $15.95 ... Hardcover $25.95

CHRONIC FATIGUE SYNDROME, FIBROMYALGIA, AND OTHER INVISIBLE ILLNESSES: A Comprehensive and Compassionate Guide *by* Katrina Berne, Ph.D.

A new edition of the classic work *Running on Empty,* this greatly revised and expanded book has the latest findings on chronic fatigue syndrome and comprehensive information about fibromyalgia, a related condition. Overlapping diseases such as environmental illness, breast implant inflammatory syndrome, lupus, Sjogren's syndrome, and post-polio syndrome are also discussed. The book includes information on possible causes, symptoms, diagnostic processes, and options for treatment.

352 pages ... Paperback $15.95 ... Hardcover $25.95

All prices subject to change

CREATING EXTRAORDINARY JOY: A Guide to Authenticity, Connection, and Self-Transformation *by* Chris Alexander

Creating Extraordinary Joy takes us on a journey of personal discovery in which we become alive to who we are, where we are in life, and what we value highly. It also helps us conenct to the authenticity and true purpose of others in a condition called "synergy," where the joining of spirit and emotion between two people creates something greater than both.

Using inspirational teachings, images from nature, simple but powerful exercises, and real-life examples, Chris Alexander describes the ten steps of life mastery. Each step yields a life lesson that takes us toward the goals of deepening our passion, opening to abundance, and giving and receiving love. This inspirational guide is more than a book; it is a path to our best self.

288 pages ... Paperback $16.95 ... Hardcover $26.95

THE PLEASURE PRESCRIPTION: To Love, to Work, to Play — Life in the Balance *by* Paul Pearsall, Ph.D.

New York Times Bestseller!

This bestselling book is a prescription for stressed-out lives. Dr. Pearsall maintains that contentment, wellness, and long life can be found by devoting time to family, helping others, and slowing down to savor life's pleasures. Pearsall's unique approach draws from Polynesian wisdom and his own 25 years of psychological and medical research. For readers who want to discover a way of life that promotes healthy values and living, *The Pleasure Prescription* provides the answers.

288 pages ... Paperback $13.95 ... Hardcover $23.95

WRITING FROM WITHIN: A Guide to Creativity and Your Life Story Writing *by* Bernard Selling

Writing from Within has attracted an enthusiastic following among those wishing to write oral histories, life narratives, or autobiographies. Bernard Selling shows new and veteran writers how to free up hidden images and thoughts, employ right-brain visualization, and use language as a way to capture feelings, people, and events. The result is at once a self-help writing workbook and an exciting journey of personal discovery and creation.

320 pages ... Paperback $17.95 ... Third Edition

ORDER FORM

10% DISCOUNT on orders of $50 or more —
20% DISCOUNT on orders of $150 or more —
30% DISCOUNT on orders of $500 or more —
On cost of books for fully prepaid orders

NAME

ADDRESS

CITY/STATE   ZIP/POSTCODE

PHONE   COUNTRY (outside of U.S.)

TITLE	QTY		PRICE	TOTAL
When Parkinson's Strikes Early (paper)		@	$15.95	
When Parkinson's Strikes Early (cloth)		@	$25.95	

Prices subject to change without notice

Please list other titles below:

		@	$	
		@	$	
		@	$	
		@	$	
		@	$	
		@	$	
		@	$	

Check here to receive our book catalog ❑   FREE

Shipping Costs

First book: $3.00 by bookpost, $4.50 by UPS, Priority Mail, or to ship outside the U.S. Each additional book: $1.00
For rush orders and bulk shipments call us at (800) 266-5592

TOTAL	_____
Less discount @____%	(_____)
TOTAL COST OF BOOKS	_____
Calif. residents add sales tax	_____
Shipping & handling	_____
TOTAL ENCLOSED	_____

Please pay in U.S. funds only

❑ Check ❑ Money Order ❑ Visa ❑ MasterCard ❑ Discover

Card # _____ Exp. date _____

Signature _____

Complete and mail to:
Hunter House Inc., Publishers
PO Box 2914, Alameda CA 94501-0914
Website: www.hunterhouse.com
Orders: (800) 266-5592 or email: ordering@hunterhouse.com
Phone (510) 865-5282 Fax (510) 865-4295

WPS 8/01